REVERSING DIABETES COOKBOOK

REVERSING DIABETES COOKBOOK

More Than 200 Delicious, Healthy Recipes

JULIAN WHITAKER, M.D.
and
PEGGY DACE

WARNER BOOKS

New York   Boston

This book is not intended as a substitute for medical advice of physicians. The reader should regularly consult a physician in all matters relating to his or her health, and particularly in respect to any symptoms that may require diagnosis or medical attention.

Copyright © 2004 by Julian Whitaker, M.D.
All rights reserved.

Warner Books
Hachette Book Group USA
1271 Avenue of the Americas, New York, NY 10020

Visit our Web site at www.HachetteBookGroupUSA.com.

Printed in the United States of America

First Edition: August 2004
10 9 8 7 6 5 4 3 2

Warner Books and the "W" logo are trademarks of Time Inc. or an affiliated company. Used under license by Hachette Book Group USA, which is not affiliated with Time Warner Inc.

Library of Congress Cataloging-in-Publication Data

Whitaker, Julian M.
Reversing diabetes cookbook : more than 200 delicious, healthy recipes / Julian Whitaker.
p. cm.
ISBN 0-446-69141-0
1. Non-insulin-dependent diabetes—Diet therapy—Recipes. I. Title.

RC662.W463 2004
641.5'6314—dc22
2003059567

Book design and text composition by Stratford Publishing Services

In memory of Kevin Kelly, friend,
gourmet, and consummate host.

Contents

Contents

Acknowledgments

I want to acknowledge all the patients I've seen and treated over the years. Working with you has taught me more about how to treat diabetes than anything I learned in medical school. Thanks to Diana Baroni at Warner Books for the inspiration for this book, to Kathy Antrim and Tareth Mitch for their excellent editing, and especially to Peggy Dace for putting these recipes together.

Julian Whitaker, M.D.

Thanks to Idel Kelly, Whitaker Wellness Institute chef, for sharing her cooking expertise and to nutritionist Diane Lara for help in developing the nutritional guidelines that define these recipes. For contributing recipes to this cookbook, I want to thank Idel, Diane, my mother-in-law Elli Boyd, and my coworkers and friends Mary Fonseca, Stacey Murray, and Teresa Herring. I especially want to acknowledge Connie Whitaker, who not only shared many recipes but also her ever-present support. A special word of thanks to my sons, Bret, Brandon, and Ben, and particularly my husband Bruce Boyd, the "food critics" who tasted every one of these recipes and helped make them better. Finally, thanks to Dr. Whitaker. Your vision, courage, and sense of humor have made for thirteen always-interesting years.

Peggy Dace

Preface

In my opinion, there is something seriously wrong with medicine today. It seems that the first-line treatment for virtually every disease is a prescription drug, and diabetes is no different. We are now in the midst of what public health officials are calling an epidemic of diabetes—more than seventeen million Americans suffer with this condition. Underlying this is an epidemic of even greater proportions: nearly two-thirds of us are overweight and a third are clinically obese. Excess weight and diabetes go hand in hand, and both are generally accompanied by poor diet and inadequate exercise.

If you are diagnosed with type 2 diabetes, your physician will probably tell you to lose weight, change your diet, and start exercising. But chances are you'll also be given a prescription for a blood sugar–lowering drug. You see, it's a lot easier for your doctor to pull out the prescription pad than it is to explain the power of lifestyle change in the management of diabetes—and then provide you with the tools and support you need to make those changes.

I've been treating diabetes and other serious diseases using diet, exercise, and targeted nutritional supplements as my primary therapies for more than a quarter of a century now. I know this approach works, not only because it is backed by tens of thousands of scientific studies published in the world's most reputable medical journals, but also because I've seen overwhelmingly positive results in thousands of patients who have opted to take control of their own health by embracing these safe, inexpensive therapies.

In *Reversing Diabetes,* I outline the treatment program we use at the Whitaker Wellness Institute. It involves regular exercise, targeted nutritional supplements, noninvasive therapies to address diabetic complications—and a comprehensive diet program. *Reversing Diabetes Cookbook* picks up where *Reversing Diabetes* leaves off. Our patients are always clamoring for recipes, so we've created more than two hundred new ones that meet all the requirements of the original recipes. They help lower blood sugar, improve the cells' sensitivity to insulin, reduce excess insulin output, and facilitate weight loss. Equally important, they taste great and are easy to prepare. Even if you don't have diabetes, I suggest you adopt a diet similar to that described in this book. At the Whitaker Wellness Institute, we use this nutrient-dense, therapeutic diet for the treatment *and* prevention of not only diabetes but also heart disease, hypertension, obesity, and most degenerative conditions.

I hope you'll enjoy these new recipes but, more important, I hope you'll utilize them as a powerful therapeutic tool in your pursuit of optimal health.

To your health,
Julian Whitaker, M.D.

PART I
The Reversing Diabetes Program

Dietary Principles for Reversing Diabetes

Diabetes is a condition marked by elevations in blood sugar. Therefore, a therapeutic diet for people with diabetes is one that helps keep blood sugar levels on an even keel, and that is exactly what the recipes in this book are designed to do. But that's not all.

High levels of glucose in the blood overwhelm the kidneys' ability to reabsorb glucose, so it is excreted in the urine—along with substantial amounts of water-soluble nutrients. These nutrient losses are a significant contributor to the complications that plague so many diabetics. The recipes in this cookbook, which use vegetables, fruits, whole grains, beans, salmon, unrefined oils, and other nutrient-dense foods, will go a long way toward improving nutritional status and protecting against diabetic complications.

The foods recommended in this book also help control insulin levels, which are often elevated in people with diabetes. When cells are resistant to the signals of insulin to let glucose in, as they are in most type 2 diabetics, the pancreas responds by producing more and more insulin to clear glucose from the blood. This condition, called insulin resistance, is associated with increased risk of heart attack, hypertension, obesity, and other problems.

Final and equally important considerations in developing these recipes were taste and ease of preparation. No matter how healthy something might be, if it doesn't taste good, you aren't going to eat it. And although you want to eat right, you probably don't want to spend hours in the kitchen. Therefore, we've included a broad range of foods, cooking methods (most of them quick and easy), and types of cuisines to satisfy every taste. We've tested and retested every one of these recipes, and we hope you like them as much as we and the friends and family members who served as our "taste testers" do.

Before we dive into the recipes, let's review the principles of the diet for reversing diabetes.

Eat the Right Carbohydrates

Carbohydrate has become a dirty word in the past few years. This is nonsense. Of course, some carbohydrate-rich foods, such as breads and other products made with white flour, are bad news. But others, including vegetables, whole grains, beans, and fruits, are a very important part of a therapeutic diabetic diet. It all depends on how a particular carbohydrate is metabolized in the body.

Although all carbs are ultimately broken down into glucose and other simple sugars, the rate at which this happens varies. Some cause a rapid and dramatic rise in blood sugar levels, while others are digested more slowly and their sugars are released into the bloodstream more gradually. Several factors determine where a food falls in this spectrum, including the type of carbohydrate and amount of fiber it contains, how much it has been processed, how long it is cooked, even how acidic it is.

Researchers have devised a means of evaluating this and assigned a set of values to foods called the *glycemic index*. The higher the glycemic index of a particular food, the faster and more dramatic the rise in blood sugar after eating it. The glycemic index is obviously very useful for people with diabetes. However, because it ignores the *amount* of carbohydrate in an average serving of a food, it needed a little refining. Enter *the glycemic load*. The glyce-mic load of a food takes into account both the glycemic index and the number of carbs per serving, giving us a more reasonable indi-cation of a food's impact on blood sugar.

Watermelon, for example, has a high glycemic index. However, a typical serving, because so much of it is water, contains very little carbohydrate and thus has a low glycemic load. Three-quarters of a cup of watermelon balls has fewer than nine grams of carbo-hydrate. In contrast, a bagel, which also has a high glycemic index, has forty-seven grams of carbs and therefore a high glycemic load. (You would have to eat a heck of a lot of watermelon to have the same impact on your blood sugar that a single bagel would have.) This means that watermelon, carrots, and some other high-glycemic index foods that diabetics may previously have shied away from are perfectly acceptable. It can swing the other way as well. Although pasta has a moderately low glycemic index, be-cause it is so carbohydrate-dense, it has a high glycemic load. This doesn't mean that you can't eat pasta, grains, and other dense carbs, but eat them in moderate quantities, as suggested in the recipes in this book. And check your blood sugar levels—some people tol-erate more carbs than others. If breads, grains, pasta, beans, and other dense carbohydrates cause problems with blood sugar con-trol, eat them less frequently and in smaller portions. (For more information on the glycemic index/load, visit Rick Mendosa's very informative Web site, www.mendosa.com.)

Glycemic index and glycemic load, of course, aren't the only considerations when selecting carbohydrate foods. Even though white sugar only has a moderately high glycemic index, it is devoid of nutrients, high in calories, and has no place in a healthy diet. In summary, minimally processed, fiber-rich, nutrient-dense, low-glycemic index vegetables, fruits, beans, and whole grains are your ticket to good blood sugar control, and they should be a founda-tion of your diet.

Adequate Protein Prevents Low Blood Sugar

It is important that everyone gets adequate amounts of protein, for the amino acids into which protein is broken down are used by the body to synthesize proteins for cellular repair and growth, as well as functional proteins like enzymes and hemoglobin. For people with diabetes, it is important for other reasons as well. Unlike carbohydrate, protein doesn't cause an immediate elevation in blood sugar, so replacing fast-burning carbohydrate with protein helps with blood sugar control. However, protein can raise blood sugar several hours after eating, as some amino acids are converted in the liver into glucose.

This is good, for it prevents between-meal hypoglycemia, or low blood sugar, which, if low enough, can be quite serious. Even if it's not life-threatening, hypoglycemia can make you tired, unfocused, irritable, and shaky. It also makes you ravenously hungry, and this is when you reach for chocolate, pretzels, and other high-glycemic carbs that quickly restore blood sugar levels.

We suggest that you eat some protein with every meal and snack, but select your protein sources wisely. Avoid saturated fat laden red meat, eat whole eggs only occasionally, and concentrate on fish, skinless poultry, low-fat dairy products, and protein-rich beans, legumes, soybeans, and tofu. (*Note:* If you have kidney disease, you'll need to cut back on your protein intake.)

Good Fats, Bad Fats

Dietary fat doesn't affect blood sugar one way or the other, so you may think that it doesn't matter how much fat you eat. Think again. Eating excesses of fat indirectly affects blood sugar control because it interferes with the actions of insulin and makes it less effective in clearing glucose out of the blood.

We're not suggesting that you eat a very low-fat diet—fat is a vital dietary component. But it is important to eat the right types of fats. Excessive intake of saturated fat found in red meat, butter, whole milk, and egg yolks raises levels of harmful LDL cholesterol and increases risk of heart disease and stroke. Occasional intake is fine, but don't make these items a daily habit. Stay completely away from trans fatty acids, which are found extensively in partially hydrogenated fats and in fried and commercially baked foods. These unnatural fats are much worse than saturated fats, for they also lower protective HDL cholesterol.

On the other hand, monounsaturated fats in olive oil, avocados, almonds, and other nuts actually protect against cardiovascular disease. And the polyunsaturated essential fatty acids in fish oils, nuts, and unprocessed vegetable oils have a multitude of health benefits. Enjoy these healthful fats, but don't go overboard, especially if you're trying to lose weight, for they are quite calorie intense.

Do Not Overeat

Not everyone with type 2 diabetes is overweight, but most are. The primary reason people gain weight is because they take in more calories than they expend. And the leading reason for this, lack of exercise notwithstanding, is because we're eating more than ever.

Researchers at New York University recently looked at the average portion sizes served today and compared them to those of several years ago, as well as to the United States Department of Agriculture standards. They found that across the board, serving sizes have ballooned—and they dramatically exceed what the USDA has established as average portions. From hamburgers and French fries to soft drinks and beer, "supersize" is all the rage. And it goes beyond fast food. Today's typical bagel is almost twice as big as the standard serving size set by the USDA, muffins are more than three times larger—and servings of pasta are almost five times heftier.

We urge you to heed the serving sizes in the recipes. If you compare the amounts of food we recommend to what you would get in a restaurant, you may think they are skimpy servings indeed. Yet they meet or exceed recommended portions. If you're still hungry, fuel up on salad, vegetables, and lean protein. Do not increase your portion sizes of starchy carbs such as pasta and bread. Better yet, eat moderately at meals and enjoy between-meal snacks, which encourage better blood sugar control. (For more on snacking, see below.)

Here are some visual size guidelines to help you estimate appropriate serving sizes:

Fish, chicken, or meat: 3 to 4 ounces = a deck of cards
Cheese: 1 ounce = a domino
Cooked pasta, rice, and beans: ½ cup = half a baseball
Raw vegetables: 1 cup = a baseball
Fruit: medium piece = a tennis ball
Dried fruit: ¼ cup = a golf ball

In Praise of Snacking

If you're like most people, you eat two or three big meals a day, not necessarily when you're hungry but when the clock says it's time to eat. Most of us work, so we're unable to disregard the clock completely. However, you can return to a more natural, healthier way of eating by partaking moderately at meals and having small snacks between meals.

We evolved as grazers, nibbling our way through the day. The natural time to eat is when you're hungry—and only enough to leave you satiated. This is particularly important for people who have diabetes. Eating smaller, more frequent meals promotes better blood sugar control, and this is especially true if those meals and snacks consist of reasonable amounts of low-glycemic carbohydrates, protein, and healthful fats. These foods fill you up and tide you over. You will feel more satiated throughout the day and have fewer blood sugar swings.

In addition to your regular meals, you should eat a small snack mid-morning, mid-afternoon, and before bedtime. Recent research suggests that a protein snack at bedtime helps maintain adequate blood sugar levels through the night. The ideal snack should be similar to the ideal meal, only smaller. Don't forget, healthy snacking also means eating less at meals. Eating snacks on top of high-calorie meals is a ticket for weight gain.

Leftovers are perfect snacks. A small serving of most any of the main dishes or soups in this cookbook makes an ideal snack. Other recipes are worth making just to have on hand for snacks.

MAKE-AHEAD SNACKS

Oatmeal Breakfast Cake: *Cakelike squares of sweetened oatmeal that you can eat at room temperature or heat for a few seconds in a microwave.* (page 44)

Apricot-Oat Granola Bars: *Cookielike and chewy, easy to tuck into a bag or lunch box.* (page 50)

Blueberry, Applesauce, and Oat Bran–Apricot Muffins: *These recipes make twelve; reheat leftovers for a snack.* (pages 48, 52, and 45)

Catalina Crab Dip: *Eat with raw vegetables.* (page 71)

Chicken and Wild Rice Salad and Chicken-Grape Salad: *Pull out a small serving of these cold chicken salads between meals.* (pages 117 and 119)

Texas Caviar: *Down-home black-eyed pea salad.* (page 133)

Falafel Sandwiches with Garlic Sauce: *Have falafel patties without the bread.* (page 106)

Crispy Cookie Bars: *Sesame seeds and oatmeal keep these cookies healthy.* (page 310)

THINGS YOU CAN QUICKLY
THROW TOGETHER IN THE KITCHEN

Cheese "Danish": *The combination of cottage cheese, fruit and sprouted-grain bread makes this a complete snack.* (page 47)

Cinnamon-Applesauce Toast: *Heated under the broiler until bubbly and warm.* (page 46)

Tutti-Frutti, Purple Haze, and Peach Smoothies: *Protein powder raises these fruit drinks a notch.* (pages 31, 30, and 80)

Nutty Breakfast Ambrosia: *A delicious combo of fruit, nuts, and yogurt.* (page 32)

Creamy Smoked Salmon: *Great on a slice of toasted rye bread.* (page 72)

Brandon's Bean Dip: *Beans, salsa, and cheese—wrap some in a tortilla.* (page 61)

Spicy Hummus: *Eat this garbanzo bean spread on pita bread.* (page 58)

Zesty Cottage Cheese: *A yummy combination of cottage cheese, radishes, onions, and green chiles.* (page 122)

HALF OF ANY ONE OF THESE
QUICK AND EASY SANDWICHES

Smoked Salmon Sandwiches (page 101)

Chicken-Chile Quesadillas (page 108)

Smart Hot Dogs (page 112)

Gourmet PB&Js (page 103)

Southwest Wraps (page 98)

Crunchy Tuna Sandwiches (page 99)

Chicken Caesar Salad Wraps (page 95)

OTHER SNACK IDEAS

Nuts and seeds: *2 tablespoons of raw almonds, sunflower seeds, pumpkin seeds, and other nuts and seeds*

Apples and nut butter: *A small sliced apple with a tablespoon of almond butter*

Cottage cheese: *Nonfat or low-fat, ½ to ¾ cup*

Yogurt: *Nonfat plain yogurt, ¾ cup, with a little stevia- or xylitol-sweetened fruit*

Turkey on rye: *A slice of turkey or chicken on a RyKrisp cracker*

Fruit and nuts: *A small piece, plus 1 tablespoon of nuts*

Edamame: *½ cup of boiled soybeans in their pods*

Whitaker Wellness Health & Nutrition Bar: *See "Resources" for details on this healthy, low-glycemic snack bar*

A One-Week Menu Plan

Sitting down once a week and planning what you're going to eat during that week saves a lot of bother, frustration, and time. No more gazing into the open fridge or freezer, hoping for an inspiration for the night's dinner. No more starting to cook a recipe, only to realize that you don't have all the ingredients. No more multiple trips to the store to purchase forgotten items.

Planning your lunches, snacks, and other meals eaten away from home is particularly important, or you'll catch yourself eating out more often than not and grabbing whatever snack you can get your hands on. Leftovers and the sandwich and soup recipes make particularly good lunches, but if they aren't available to reheat or fix in a hurry, you're not going to bother. It seems as if we're always in a rush in the morning, so we've found that preparing the next day's lunch the evening before is the best way to go. Another suggestion is to make double batches of your favorite soup or main dish recipes on the weekend and freeze individual-sized portions. Then all you'll have to do is pop them into the microwave.

It takes some time and discipline to get into the habit of menu planning, but it truly is worth it. The following is a sample one-week menu plan, including snacks, to give you an idea of how to put meals together.

Day 1

Breakfast
Breakfast Burrito (page 38)
Quick and Easy Salsa
    (page 284)
Whole orange
Cup of coffee

Morning Snack
Apricot-Oat Granola Bar
    (page 50)

Lunch
Crunchy Tuna Sandwich
    (page 99)
Granny's Apples (page 302)

Afternoon Snack
Creamy Smoked Salmon
    (page 72)
3 rye crackers

Dinner
Lasagna Roll-Ups (page 223)
Orange County Special
    (page 130)
Apple-Pear Crisp (page 313)

Evening Snack
Purple Haze Smoothie
    (page 30)

Day 2

Breakfast
Nutty Breakfast Ambrosia
    (page 32)
Slice of sprouted-grain bread
Cup of tea

Morning Snack
Blueberry Muffin (page 48)

Lunch
BLT Salad (page 116)
Gourmet PB&J (page 103)

Afternoon Snack
Whole apple
¼ cup almonds

Dinner
Easy Baked Barbecue
    Chicken (page 171)
Sweet Potato Salad (page 135)
Louisiana-Style Greens
    (page 252)
Blueberry Crumble
    (page 314)

Evening Snack
¾ cup fat-free cottage cheese

Day 3

Breakfast
Basic Whole Grain Cereal
(page 33)
¾ cup skim milk
½ cup blueberries
Cup of coffee

Morning Snack
Chicken-Grape Salad
(page 119)
½ slice of sprouted-grain
bread

Lunch
Chipotle Chili (page 140)
3 whole wheat crackers

Afternoon Snack
Peach Smoothie (page 80)

Dinner
Teriyaki Salmon (page 198)
Sesame Green Beans
(page 256)
Thai Noodles (page 272)

Evening Snack
1 cup nonfat plain yogurt
½ pear
Stevia

Day 4

Breakfast
The Perfect Omelet (page 35)
Healthy Home Fries
(page 41)
Cup of coffee

Morning Snack
Cinnamon-Applesauce Toast
(page 46)

Lunch
Chicken Caesar Salad Wrap
(page 95)
Cream of Broccoli Soup
(page 163)

Afternoon Snack
Spicy Hummus (page 58)
½ whole wheat pita bread
round

Dinner
Two-Hour Roasted Turkey
(page 187)
Pecan Stuffing (page 269)
Gravy (page 293)
Zucchini-Leek Sauté
(page 259)

Evening Snack
Crispy Cookie Bar (page 310)

Day 5

Breakfast
Cheese "Danish"
    (page 47)
Tutti-Frutti Smoothie
    (page 31)
Cup of coffee

Morning Snack
¼ pumpkin seeds
¼ dried apricots

Lunch
Grandma's Vegetable-Beefy
    Stew (page 157)
1 ounce low-sodium cheese
3 rye crackers

Afternoon Snack
2 ounces turkey slices
Slice of sprouted-grain bread
2 slices fresh tomato

Dinner
Scampi in Wine and Garlic
    Sauce (page 216)
Broccoli with Lemon-Chive
    Sauce (page 260)
Wild Rice and Mushroom
    Medley (page 264)

Evening Snack
1 cup nonfat plain yogurt
½ cup raspberries
Stevia

Day 6

Breakfast
Confetti Egg White Scramble
    (page 37)
Slice of sprouted-grain bread
½ cup strawberries
Cup of coffee

Morning Snack
Orange Slush (page 79)
Applesauce Muffin (page 52)

Lunch
Mexican Pizza (page 249)
Mary's Fresh Salsa (page 283)
Tex-Mex Corn Salad
    (page 134)

Afternoon Snack
Emerald Dip (page 62)
1 stalk celery, sliced lengthwise
1 medium carrot, sliced
    lengthwise

Dinner
Crispy Chicken Tenders
    (page 174)
Luscious Layered Salad
    (page 120)
Roasted Winter Vegetables
    (page 257)

Evening Snack
Apple-Pear Crisp (page 313)

Day 7

Breakfast
Oatmeal Griddle Cakes
   (page 43)
1 whole pear
Virgin Bloody Mary (page 84)

Morning Snack
Oatmeal Breakfast Cake
   (page 44)
Sugar-Free Lemonade
   (page 81)

Lunch
Shrimp Louie (page 121)
4 whole wheat crackers

Afternoon Snack
Peach Smoothie (page 80)

Dinner
Lemon-Mustard Chicken
   Breasts (page 193)
Grilled Pesto Vegetables
   (page 253)
Quinoa Pilaf (page 268)
Blue Cheese Lovers' Salad
   (page 125)

Evening Snack
¾ cup nonfat cottage cheese

The Healthy Kitchen

Here is some basic information about the ingredients used in this cookbook. You should be able to find almost everything in your grocery store; the few exceptions are available in most health food stores or they can also be ordered. (See "Resources" on page 323.)

Kitchen Equipment

You probably already have most everything you'll need in your kitchen: good knives, a cutting board, wooden spoons, a wire whisk, measuring cups and spoons, and assorted baking dishes and saucepans. One inexpensive kitchen gadget we do recommend is a garlic press. You will also need nonstick skillets to cut down on the amount of fat you need to sauté vegetables and other foods. Several recipes require a blender or food processor, and a few call for a microwave. You can do without the microwave—we don't use it for much except heating things and steaming vegetables. If you have an outdoor grill and/or a George Foreman grill, you'll find yourself using it often, but it isn't a necessity.

Oils

You'll see extra-virgin olive oil in a lot of our recipes. Olive oil (make sure it's extra-virgin) is a heart-healthy monounsaturated oil. It can tolerate moderate heat, but don't heat it over high heat.

Other good monounsaturated oils, which are especially nice when you don't want the strong flavor of olive oil, include hazelnut, almond, avocado, and, when you want an Asian flavor, sesame oil. (We're not crazy about canola because it is highly processed.) You'll also use a lot of olive oil spray to coat skillets and baking pans. You may want to purchase an oil mister and fill it with olive, almond, or avocado oil.

Expeller-pressed, minimally processed polyunsaturated oils, such as those from grape seeds, sunflower seeds, sesame seeds, and walnuts, have health benefits, but they are not appropriate for cooking. Polyunsaturated oils are very fragile and break down into free radicals and other undesirable by-products when heated. Use them in salad dressings, if desired, or add them after dishes are cooked. You'll find expeller-pressed mono- and polyunsaturated oils in your health food store. Buy brands that are packed in dark bottles, and store them in the refrigerator. Our favorite brand is Omega Nutrition.

A few of our recipes call for butter, and organic is preferable. We do not recommend margarines, for almost all of them contain at least some partially hydrogenated oils. If you feel the need for a bread spread use butter or mix equal parts of butter and olive oil.

Sweeteners

A little sugar of any kind isn't going to hurt anyone, but everyone and especially diabetics need to be smart about sweeteners. In addition to honey (which we use in only one recipe), here are the healthy sweeteners we use in this book. (If you can't find these in your health food store, see "Resources" for ordering information.)

Xylitol: Extracted from birch trees and corncobs, xylitol looks and tastes similar to white sugar (it's lighter and fluffier). This makes it an ideal substitute for sugar in baking and other recipes. Although xylitol is not calorie-free, it is very slowly metabolized and has a very low glycemic index. It's a little pricey, but you're not going to be using too much of it.

Stevia: An herbal sweetener from *Stevia rebaudiana,* a plant native to South America, stevia comes in both unrefined extracts and refined, concentrated liquids and powders. Our favorite for cooking is the refined clear liquid extract. The powder is acceptable, but it's easier to squeeze a few drops out of an eyedropper or bottle than to measure the powdered extract. Be careful when you use stevia—it is 200 to 250 times sweeter than sugar, and if you use too much, it has a rather strong aftertaste. If you've tried stevia and didn't like it, try using less, or experiment with another brand, for some have more of an aftertaste than others.

Brown Rice Syrup: Thick and syrupy, brown rice syrup has a stronger taste than honey. It is very slowly metabolized, so it causes no dramatic rises in blood sugar. Brown rice syrup makes a nice topping for French toast, pancakes, and hot cereal. It may also be used in recipes that call for honey.

We do not recommend the artificial sweetener aspartame (Nutrasweet and Equal) for it is metabolized into several toxic by-products and has been linked to headaches, seizures, mood disorders, vision problems, and brain tumors. Nor can we recommend other artificial sweeteners—there just isn't enough research to prove their safety. We also recommend staying away from fructose as an added sweetener, especially in the form of high-fructose corn syrup. Even though it has a very low glycemic index and doesn't affect blood sugar much, excessive amounts raise fatty acid and triglyceride levels and interfere with insulin sensitivity. Excesses also contribute to elevated blood pressure and cholesterol, which plague many diabetics.

Salt and Salt Substitutes

Many people who have diabetes also have hypertension because insulin resistance is an underlying factor in both conditions. Even if your blood pressure is in the normal range, we suggest that you monitor your sodium intake—and not just for the sake of your blood pressure. High intake of sodium is also associated with increased risk of osteoporosis (it leaches calcium out of the bones), ulcers, and stomach cancer.

Since sodium is ubiquitous in even minimally processed foods such as canned tomatoes and beans, always shop for low-sodium varieties. Soup stock or broth is another high-sodium item we use often in these recipes, so you'll need to find low-sodium brands.

We do call for a little salt or seasoned salt in many recipes, and we always give the option of salt substitute. Nu-Salt (potassium chloride) contains no sodium and 528 milligrams of potassium per ⅛ teaspoon. Although some people find that it has a slightly metallic taste, for most it is a fine substitute for salt. Another option is Cardia Salt, which is a combination of sodium (135 mg per ⅛ teaspoon), potassium (90 mg), and a little magnesium and l-lysine. Seasoned salt like Lowry's provides more flavor with less sodium. Try our Low-Sodium Seasoned Salt (page 297)—we think it's quite good.

Go as low as you can, but don't fret about every milligram of sodium, for it is balanced by the large amounts of potassium you'll be getting in all the plant foods you eat on this diet.

Baking Staples

Cornstarch or arrowroot, baking soda, baking powder, and whole wheat flour are must-haves. Stone-ground whole wheat flour is the most healthful but also the graniest and heaviest. Whole wheat pastry flour, which is more finely ground, or unbleached white flour yields better results in some recipes, as indicated. Because whole wheat flour, unlike white flour, contains natural oils, it is prone to rancidity. Store it tightly sealed in the freezer. You may also want to experiment with spelt, barley, and amaranth flours, although we don't call for them in this cookbook.

Herbs and Seasonings

There's nothing like an assortment of fresh herbs to season your food. Most grocery stores carry fresh herbs, and you should also consider growing your own herbs, either in your garden or in pots in your kitchen. Always have fresh parsley and cilantro on hand, for they are ingredients in many of these recipes. You can dramatically extend cilantro's rather short shelf life by placing the stems in a mug half filled with water (as you'd place flowers in a vase) and loosely covering the leaves with a plastic bag.

We also use a lot of fresh garlic. When we call for a clove of garlic, use a medium-sized clove. (Some cloves are colossal!) Store fresh garlic in a dark, cool area that allows circulation of air—not in the fridge or a plastic bag. Garlic and onion powder (not salt) are also handy to have around. A garlic press, which minces the garlic for you, is an essential kitchen tool.

Dried herbs are also wonderful, and we recommend that you keep a variety on hand. Some of the seasonings we call for include freshly ground black pepper, cumin, coriander, ginger, oregano, basil, thyme, crushed red pepper flakes, cayenne, curry powder, dried chives, chili powder, and cinnamon. Sodium-free herbal blends we use include Italian seasoning and Mrs. Dash seasoning blend. You should have vanilla extract as well.

Dried Beans, Grains, Pasta, and Cereals

Our recipes call for the following types of beans and whole grains: lentils, garbanzo beans, white beans, kidney beans, bulgur, quinoa, pearl barley, and long-grain brown rice. To save time, we often suggest using canned beans.

Pastas to keep in your cupboard include couscous, spaghetti, lasagna, linguine, elbow macaroni, and angel hair pasta. Also, look for high-protein pasta, which is becoming more and more popular. (See Resources section.)

The cereal we use most often is rolled oats (long-cooking oatmeal), along with oat bran and, in a couple of recipes, Kellogg's Special K cereal to coat fish and chicken before baking. Any whole grain can be eaten as hot cereal (see page 33 for details). The only cold cereals with a glycemic index low enough for us to recommend to people with diabetes are those made with 100 percent bran.

Nuts and Seeds

Purchase raw almonds, pumpkin seeds, sunflower seeds, flaxseeds, and sesame seeds and store them in your freezer. (You don't have to freeze flaxseeds since their protective outer coat is intact.)

Breads

Sprouted-grain bread, which is made without flour, and dark whole-grain pumpernickel and rye breads have the lowest glycemic index and are therefore the best for diabetics. Some good brands of sprouted-grain breads include French Meadow Bakery, Food For Life (which makes Ezekiel bread), and Trader Joe's (found only in Trader Joe's stores). Whole wheat pita and whole wheat tortillas are acceptable in moderation. Because of its acidity, sourdough bread also has a fairly low glycemic index, but we don't recommend it very often because it lacks the nutritional value of whole-grain bread. You're not going to be eating a whole lot of bread, and natural breads don't have a very long shelf life. Store them in the freezer.

The best crackers are those made with coarse flour, and even they have a moderately high glycemic index, so eat them in moderation. Suggested brands include Ak-Mak 100 percent whole wheat crackers, Ryvita, and RyKrisp bread.

Fresh and Frozen Fruits and Vegetables

Fresh produce always has the best texture and taste. Take advantage of some of the shortcuts now appearing in the produce section: cleaned spinach and other greens, peeled baby carrots, bags of mixed salad greens, and fresh herbs. We are big fans of all of these, especially rinsed greens, which can be a bear to clean.

If you can find organic produce, go for it. Regulations defining exactly what organic means are finally in place, so you can rest assured that you are getting cleaner, fresher, environmentally friendlier food. You still need to wash organic fruits and vegetables, as you would any produce.

Some of the fresh fruits and vegetables we suggest you always keep on hand include onions, apples, oranges, lemons, limes, lettuce, tomatoes, and parsley. You'll be using these often, and they keep pretty well. If you have other favorites, of course you'll want to keep them on hand. Purchase additional produce as you plan to use it.

Believe it or not, frozen produce is as nutritious as fresh, although taste and particularly texture sometimes suffer during processing. Our favorite frozen veggies include green peas, corn, chopped or sliced bell peppers, chopped spinach, and greens such as mustard and kale. Get the large, one-pound bags so you can use what you need, then reseal them. Similar bags of frozen blue-berries, strawberries, raspberries, and peaches should also be kept around. Stay away from small boxes of fruit frozen in syrup—they contain too much sugar.

Canned Vegetables and Fruits

We make liberal use of canned tomatoes, tomato sauce, and tomato paste (low-sodium or salt-free varieties) as well as canned beans. If you have a favorite low-fat, low-sodium spaghetti sauce, feel free to use it. Canned beans to keep in your pantry include garbanzos, kidney beans, pinto beans, and black-eyed peas. Before using canned beans, pour them into a colander, rinse well under running water to remove excess sodium, and drain. Canned ripe olives and mild chopped green chiles are also used fairly often.

Juices

A few recipes call for small amounts of frozen apple or orange juice concentrate as a sweetener, but even in the beverage section, you won't see many fruit juice recipes—whole fruit in smoothies, but not fruit juice. Although fruit juice contains many of the same antioxidants and protective phytonutrients as whole fruit, it loses much of its fiber, which slows the release of sugar into the bloodstream.

Miscellaneous Prepared Foods

Miscellaneous canned and prepared foods frequently used in these recipes include evaporated low-fat or fat-free milk, low-fat or fat-free mayonnaise, salsa, low-sodium soy sauce, vinegar (balsamic, rice, and red wine vinegar), bottled lemon and lime juice (as a backup), Tabasco sauce, ketchup (low-sodium, low-sugar), and Dijon mustard.

We use a lot of chicken or vegetarian broth or stock. You may use canned broth or bouillon cubes, but make sure you search out low-sodium varieties, for these pack a punch of salt. You may have to check your health food store. Also keep natural-style peanut butter (without hydrogenated oils) and tahini (sesame butter) in stock.

Dairy and Eggs

Nonfat plain yogurt is a recurring ingredient in this cookbook. So is low-fat or nonfat cottage cheese. We occasionally call for low-fat or nonfat ricotta cheese, sour cream, and evaporated milk, as well as skim buttermilk. Cheeses used include Parmesan (freshly grated in the cheese section is much better than that in the tall cans you'll find in the spaghetti sauce aisle), low-sodium Cheddar, and occasionally feta and Swiss.

We also use a lot of egg whites (the yolks are discarded in almost all of the recipes). An option, and one we prefer, is Egg Beaters, an egg white product that is 99 percent egg whites with a little yellow coloring. ReddiEggs and Second Nature Eggs—also egg white products—work well, too. They keep well in the refrigerator, and you won't miss breaking and separating eggs. A quarter cup equals one egg. If you buy whole eggs, purchase large, free-range eggs.

Poultry, Fish, and Soy Protein

You'll see a lot of chicken breasts in the recipes. A huge time-saver is to purchase large bags of frozen, skinned, boned breasts. Pull out as many as you need and defrost them overnight in the fridge or more quickly in the microwave. Keeping lean ground turkey in your freezer is also advisable. Free-range chickens are pricier, but they're raised in much more humane conditions and are free of the antibiotics and hormones most chickens are given.

Fresh seafood is best, but frozen is a reasonable substitute. We especially like bags of shelled, deveined, and cleaned raw shrimp. Take out what you need, defrost under cold running water, and it's ready to cook. Bags of ready-to-cook fish fillets are another nice shortcut. Canned water-packed tuna (albacore has the best texture), salmon, and clams are also used in a few recipes. You have to be careful about what species of fish you eat these days, for large, long-lived predatory species may harbor unsafe levels of mercury. The fish we call for in this cookbook, such as salmon, shrimp, halibut, and mahi-mahi, are all considered safe. We use canned tuna in a couple of recipes, but you shouldn't eat more than a can a week. Wild Pacific salmon is preferable to farm-raised Atlantic salmon (wild Atlantic salmon is very rare these days). Farmed salmon may be exposed to antibiotics, pesticides, and pigments (to achieve the characteristic color)—and many consider them a threat to the environment and to wild salmon.

Don't shy away from trying the recipes that include tofu and other soy products, such as the "hamburgers" and "hot dogs" on pages 109 and 112. They are amazingly good.

Beverages, Alcoholic and Other

The beverage recipes in the cookbook are a mixed lot and contain ingredients that you wouldn't necessarily need to have as kitchen staples. We suggest keeping black, herbal, and especially green tea on hand, as well as coffee to use in moderation. We don't call for a lot of juice but do use low-sodium V8 juice and orange juice occasionally. We have included two alcoholic drink recipes, and a few of our other recipes call for wine or liqueur, which may be omitted, if desired.

Enjoy This Cookbook

We've tried to make this cookbook as user friendly as possible. Most recipes make four servings, although some serve six or more and a few serve just two. In addition to the recipes, we've included yields, times, serving suggestions, health tips, and cooks' notes with every recipe.

We have also provided a nutritional analysis with each recipe, which includes basic information such as calories, carbohydrates, fat, protein, and sodium, as well as diabetic exchanges, for those who are interested. Nutritional information was calculated using MasterCook software (ValuSoft, Inc., 711 S. Pine St., Waconia, MN 55387). We have spot-checked these calculations against other software, as well as USDA nutritional charts, and found them to be quite accurate. Our apologies for any errors that may appear in these analyses.

PART II
Recipes

———————

Breakfast

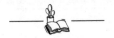

Adelle Davis, one of the earliest food gurus, once said, "Eat break-fast like a king, lunch like a prince, and dinner like a pauper." This is good advice, but most people ignore it. When you wake up in the morning, your energy stores are low, so naturally you should eat a good breakfast. Unfortunately, this most important meal is the one that many people leave by the wayside. "I'm not hungry in the morning." "I don't have time to fix breakfast." Or they eat a bowl of cold cereal with a sky-high glycemic index. Either way, they set into motion a cycle of blood sugar swings that may last throughout the day.

Make a point to eat breakfast every day, and select breakfast foods that don't drive your blood sugar rapidly up but provide a slow and sustained release of glucose, such as oatmeal and other whole-grain cereals, egg whites, and fruit-sweetened yogurt. We know you don't have time most mornings to labor in the kitchen, so we've intentionally kept the bulk of the recipes in this chapter quick and simple. If you really have a problem eating breakfast, try the smoothie recipes for a hearty breakfast on the run.

Purple Haze Smoothie

Frozen berries make this colorful, quick, and easy.

MAKES 2 SERVINGS (2½ CUPS)   PREPARATION TIME: 10 MINUTES

1½ cups water
¼   cup freshly ground flaxseeds
1   scoop protein powder
¾   cup frozen blueberries
¾   cup frozen strawberries
6   drops stevia, or to taste

Place water, flaxseed, and protein powder in blender. While blender is running, add frozen berries, a few at a time. Process until smooth and creamy, adding more water if needed to achieve desired consistency. Add stevia, 2 drops at a time, to taste.

PER SERVING: 194 calories; 8 g fat (35% calories from fat); 14 g protein (The protein content will vary according to the type of protein powder you use. We used Designer Whey Protein.); 19 g carbohydrate; 8 g dietary fiber; 15 mg cholesterol; 33 mg sodium. EXCHANGES: ½ grain (starch); 1½ lean meat; 1 fruit; 1 fat.

SERVING IDEAS: Any frozen fruit will work in this recipe. If you use fresh fruit, substitute half of the water with ice. For added nutrition, add a scoop of Essential Greens or another dehydrated "green drink" powder. You'll find many good brands in your health food store.

Tutti-Frutti Smoothie

A quick, nutritious drink.

MAKES 2 SERVINGS (2½ CUPS)   PREPARATION TIME: 10 MINUTES

1 *cup water*
¼ *cup freshly ground flaxseeds*
1 *scoop protein powder*
1 *barely ripe banana*
1 *orange, peeled*
½ *cup ice cubes*
4 *drops stevia, or to taste*

Place water, flaxseed, and protein powder in blender. With blender running, add banana, orange, and ice. Blend until smooth, adding more water or ice as needed to attain desired thickness. Add stevia, 2 drops at a time, to taste.

PER SERVING: 230 calories; 8 g fat (28.5% calories from fat); 14 g protein; 29 g carbohydrate; 8 g dietary fiber; 15 mg cholesterol; 32 mg sodium. EXCHANGES: ½ grain (starch); 1½ lean meat; 1½ fruit; 1 fat.

SERVING IDEAS: Variations on this smoothie recipe are endless. You can use any type of fresh or frozen fruit. (If the fruit is frozen, omit the ice.) You can also use soy milk or skim milk in place of water, if desired.

Note
Bananas, especially ripe ones, have a high glycemic index. Eat them sparingly, and only when they're just barely ripe. If uneaten bananas get too ripe, peel them, wrap in plastic, and freeze for later use in smoothies.

Nutty Breakfast Ambrosia

High in protein, healthful fats, vitamins, and minerals—
and your favorite fruit.

MAKES 4 SERVINGS (3 CUPS)   PREPARATION TIME: 10 MINUTES

2 *cups fruit (any single or mixed fruit of your choice),*
   chopped or sliced
¼ *cup raw almonds, chopped*
¼ *cup raw sunflower seeds*
¼ *cup raw pumpkin seeds, roasted*
1½ *cups nonfat plain yogurt*
10 *drops stevia or 1 tablespoon xylitol, or to taste*

Mix fruit, nuts, and seeds in a medium bowl. Fold in yogurt and stir
well. Add stevia, 1 drop at a time, or xylitol, 1 teaspoon at a time,
stir, and taste. Add more, by the drop or teaspoonful, as desired.

PER SERVING: 204 calories; 10 g fat (42.9% calories from fat); 10 g
protein; 21 g carbohydrate; 4 g dietary fiber; 2 mg cholesterol; 67
mg sodium. EXCHANGES: ½ grain (starch); ½ lean meat; ½ fruit; ½
nonfat milk; 1½ fat.

SERVING IDEAS: This combination of yogurt, fruit, nuts, and seeds is
extremely versatile. Use your favorite fruit (limit to ½ to 1 cup of
fruit per person) and nuts, and experiment with different sweeteners: stevia, xylitol, brown rice syrup, or a small amount of fruit
juice-sweetened jam.

Note

If you're not crazy about yogurt, especially unsweetened yogurt,
try other brands until you find one you like. Each has a distinct
taste, depending on the cultures used to ferment it.

Basic Whole Grain Cereal

Start your day with the goodness of whole grains.

3 *cups water*
1 *cup 7-grain cereal or other whole grains (see Notes)*
1 *cup skim milk or soy milk*
1 *cup chopped peaches or other fruit*
8 *drops stevia, or to taste*

Bring water to a boil, add cereal, reduce heat, and cover. Cook for 10 to 15 minutes until tender.

Transfer to serving bowls and top each serving with ¼ cup each of milk and fruit. Sweeten with stevia to taste.

PER SERVING: 146 calories; 2 g fat (8.9% calories from fat); 7 g protein; 31 g carbohydrate; 6 g dietary fiber; 1 mg cholesterol; 37 mg sodium. EXCHANGES: 1½ grain (starch); ½ fruit; ½ fat.

SERVING IDEA: Another great topping for hot cereal (per serving): ¼ cup chopped dried apricots, ¼ cup chopped almonds, and ⅛ teaspoon almond extract.

Note

Try these other whole grains for breakfast. Here are approximate amount of water and cooking time per cup of cereal: whole wheat and whole rye, 2½ cups water, 1 hour; pearl barley, 3 cups water, 50 minutes; flaked wheat or rye, 2 cups water, 20 minutes; steel-cut oats, 3 cups water, 30 minutes; quinoa, 2 cups water, 15 minutes.

Apple Muesli

A healthy import from Switzerland.

MAKES 4 SERVINGS (2½ CUPS)   PREPARATION TIME: 4 HOURS 10 MINUTES

1   *cup old-fashioned rolled oats (preferably steel-cut)*
½   *cup skim milk*
¼   *cup chopped dried apricots*
½   *cup nonfat plain yogurt*
⅓   *cup chopped almonds*
1   *small apple, cored and grated (peeling optional)*
8   *drops stevia, or to taste*

Mix oats, milk, and apricots together, cover, and refrigerate for at least 4 hours, or overnight.

Stir in yogurt, almonds, apple, and stevia, to taste. Mix well and serve.

PER SERVING: 217 calories; 8 g fat (31% calories from fat); 9 g protein; 30 g carbohydrate; 5 g dietary fiber; 1 mg cholesterol; 45 mg sodium. EXCHANGES: 1 grain (starch); ½ lean meat; ½ fruit; ½ nonfat milk; ½ fat.

Note

Oats are a rich source of avenanthramides, which have twice the antioxidant power of vitamin E. They also reduce cardiovascular risk by combating inflammation and slowing the process of atherosclerosis.

The Perfect Omelet

This should be in every cook's repertoire.

MAKES 1 SERVING   PREPARATION TIME: 10 MINUTES

4   egg whites or ½ cup Egg Beaters or other egg white product
    Dash salt or salt substitute
    Dash freshly ground black pepper
1   teaspoon water
½   teaspoon butter or olive oil spray

In a small bowl, beat egg whites, salt, pepper, and water with a fork until well mixed.

Heat an 8-inch nonstick skillet over medium-high heat. Add butter and swirl around until butter coats bottom of pan (or spray with olive oil spray).

Pour eggs into the skillet and slide the skillet back and forth to distribute eggs over the bottom of the skillet. As eggs begin to set, tilt the skillet and lift edge of omelet, allowing uncooked eggs on top to slide underneath. When omelet is set, let it stand over the heat for a few seconds to brown the bottom.

Slide omelet onto a plate, fill with your favorite prepared filling, fold, and serve.

PER SERVING: 84 calories; 2 g fat (21.8% calories from fat); 14 g protein; 1 g carbohydrate; 5 mg cholesterol; 239 mg sodium. EXCHANGES: 2 lean meat; ½ fat.

SERVING IDEA: Just before cooking eggs, prepare your favorite filling by sautéing in a nonstick skillet sprayed with olive oil spray: ½ cup mushrooms, onions, zucchini, spinach, asparagus, or any

(continued)

The Perfect Omelet (continued)

combination of vegetables. Place on omelet, top with 1 tablespoon grated cheese (if desired), fold, and serve.

Note

Although whole eggs—up to seven a week—are not considered to be a health risk for most people, they are a concern for diabetics, whose ability to handle cholesterol is compromised. A Harvard study has found that diabetics who eat just one egg a day have a significantly higher risk of heart disease compared to those who eat only one whole egg or less a week. Stick with egg whites—they are mostly protein and contain no cholesterol. You may add a dash of turmeric, the spice that gives curry powder its deep color, to give the eggs a hint of yellow. Or use Egg Beaters or another brand of packaged egg whites.

Confetti Egg White Scramble

*Dress up scrambled eggs with colorful,
nutritious vegetables.*

MAKES 2 SERVINGS (2 CUPS)   PREPARATION TIME: 20 MINUTES

1   *teaspoon extra-virgin olive oil*
½   *cup chopped onion*
½   *cup chopped zucchini*
½   *cup chopped red bell pepper*
8   *egg whites or 1 cup Egg Beaters or other egg white product*
1   *tablespoon water*
1   *tablespoon grated Parmesan cheese*
¼   *teaspoon freshly ground black pepper*

Heat olive oil in a medium nonstick skillet over medium-high heat.

Add onion, zucchini, and red pepper to the skillet and sauté, stirring occasionally, for 2 to 3 minutes, until tender-crisp.

Meanwhile, lightly beat egg whites, water, Parmesan cheese, and black pepper.

Pour eggs into skillet and continue to cook another 1 to 2 minutes, stirring often, until eggs are set.

PER SERVING: 128 calories; 3 g fat (22.5% calories from fat); 16 g protein; 8 g carbohydrate; 2 g dietary fiber; 2 mg cholesterol; 269 mg sodium. EXCHANGES: 2 lean meat; 1 vegetable; ½ fat.

Note
Red bell peppers have three times more vitamin C and eleven times more beta-carotene than green peppers.

Breakfast Burritos

Good for breakfast, lunch, or dinner.

 1 *teaspoon extra-virgin olive oil*
 1 *small onion, chopped*
 ½ *medium green bell pepper, chopped*
10 *egg whites or 1¼ cups Egg Beaters or other egg white product*
 ½ *cup cooked pinto beans (canned or home-cooked), rinsed and drained, or refried beans*
 4 *whole wheat tortillas*
 4 *tablespoons grated sharp Cheddar cheese*
 1 *small tomato, chopped*
 2 *green onions, thinly sliced*
 4 *tablespoons freshly chopped cilantro*

In a large nonstick skillet, heat olive oil over medium heat. Add onion and green pepper and sauté, stirring frequently, for 3 to 4 minutes. Pour in egg whites and cook, stirring occasionally, until eggs are just set, 2 to 3 minutes.

Meanwhile, heat beans in a small saucepan or in the microwave until hot.

Warm tortillas by preheating a nonstick skillet over medium heat. Place tortillas, one at a time, in the skillet and cook until hot yet still pliable, about a minute per side. Keep warm.

Spoon eggs, beans, and cheese into each tortilla. Top with tomato, green onions, and cilantro. Roll up and serve.

PER SERVING: 210 calories; 4 g fat (17% calories from fat); 16 g protein; 33 g carbohydrate; 3 g dietary fiber; 7 mg cholesterol; 361 mg sodium. EXCHANGES: 2 grain (starch); 1½ lean meat; 1 vegetable; ½ fat.

SERVING IDEA: Serve with Mary's Fresh Salsa (page 283), Quick and Easy Salsa (page 284), or store-bought salsa.

Note
Cooking a pot of beans ahead of time to have on hand for making dishes like this is a good idea. Cover beans in water, soak overnight, drain, cover again with fresh water, and simmer for 1 to 2 hours, depending on the beans. They will keep in the fridge for a week, or you can freeze them in 1-cup containers for later use.

Bombay Breakfast

Eggs with an Indian twist.

MAKES 4 SERVINGS   PREPARATION TIME: 25 MINUTES

16 egg whites or 2 cups Egg Beaters or other egg white product
¼   teaspoon salt or salt substitute
¼   teaspoon freshly ground black pepper
1   tablespoon extra-virgin olive oil
1   medium onion, chopped
¾   cup chopped mushrooms
1½ teaspoons curry powder, or more to taste
1   tomato (fresh or canned), seeded and diced
4   sprigs cilantro, for garnish

Mix eggs, salt, and pepper together in a medium bowl and stir until well blended.

In a large nonstick skillet, heat olive oil over medium heat. Add onion and cook for 5 minutes, stirring occasionally.

Add mushrooms and curry powder and cook, stirring often, for 3 more minutes. Add tomato and continue cooking, stirring frequently, for 2 more minutes.

Pour eggs into the skillet and cook, stirring constantly, just until eggs are set, 3 to 4 minutes. Do not overcook.

Garnish with cilantro.

PER SERVING: 105 calories; 2 g fat (13.1% calories from fat); 15 g protein; 7 g carbohydrate; 1 g dietary fiber; 0 mg cholesterol; 361 mg sodium. EXCHANGES: 2 lean meat; 1 vegetable.

SERVING IDEA: Serve this with chapatti (unleavened, whole wheat Indian bread), or whole wheat tortillas and Raita (page 286).

Healthy Home Fries

Made with sweet potatoes and onions.

MAKES 4 SERVINGS   PREPARATION TIME: 20 MINUTES

1   *pound (about 1½ large) sweet potatoes*
1   *cup water*
1   *teaspoon extra-virgin olive oil*
1   *large onion, chopped*
½   *teaspoon Low-Sodium Seasoned Salt (page 297) or salt substitute*
¼   *teaspoon onion powder*
¼   *teaspoon freshly ground black pepper*

Peel sweet potatoes, cut in half lengthwise, then cut halves into thin slices, about ¼ inch.

Place potatoes in a covered microwave-safe dish. Add water and cook in a microwave on high for 5 minutes, until tender. (You may also cook in a covered saucepan until tender, 5 to 10 minutes.) Drain well.

Heat olive oil in a large nonstick skillet over medium-high heat. Add potatoes, onion, and seasonings to skillet and cook, stirring often, for 5 to 6 minutes, until onion is cooked and potatoes lightly browned and tender.

PER SERVING: 108 calories; 1 g fat (11.7% calories from fat); 2 g protein; 22 g carbohydrate; 3 g dietary fiber; 0 mg cholesterol; 184 mg sodium. EXCHANGES: 1½ grain (starch); ½ vegetable.

SERVING IDEA: Serve in place of hash browns or home fries—for breakfast or anytime. Dip in ketchup, close your eyes, and you'll swear you're eating white potatoes.

(continued)

Healthy Home Fries (continued)

Note

Sweet potatoes are one of the most nutritious vegetables. A medium sweet potato contains just 130 calories, 31 grams of carbohydrate, and a trace of fat—but it packs in 3.9 grams of fiber, significant amounts of vitamin C, potassium, and calcium, and an astounding 26,081 IU of beta-carotene. Beta-carotene is a potent antioxidant and is necessary for vision, bone and tissue growth, and immune function. It helps maintain healthy skin and mucous membranes and protects against cardiovascular disease, stroke, and several types of cancer.

Oatmeal Griddle Cakes
A weekend treat.

MAKES 4 SERVINGS (8 GRIDDLE CAKES)   PREPARATION TIME: 10 MINUTES

½ cup old-fashioned rolled oats
½ cup whole wheat flour
¾ cup reduced-fat buttermilk
¼ cup skim milk
2 egg whites or ¼ cup Egg Beaters or other egg white product
1 tablespoon xylitol
2 tablespoons hazelnut oil or almond oil
1 teaspoon baking powder
½ teaspoon baking soda
¼ teaspoon salt or salt substitute
   Olive oil spray

Heat a nonstick griddle to 375 degrees F or a large nonstick skillet over medium heat.

Meanwhile, using an electric mixer or whisk, beat all ingredients except olive oil spray together just until smooth.

Spray the griddle or skillet with olive oil spray. For each griddle cake, pour ¼ cup batter onto griddle or skillet. (If batter is too thick, thin with a little milk.) Cook until griddle cakes become puffy and bubbles form on the surface, about 3 minutes. Turn, and cook the other side for another 1 to 2 minutes, until golden brown.

PER SERVING: 182 calories; 8 g fat (38.3% calories from fat); 6 g protein; 24 g carbohydrate; 3 g dietary fiber; 2 mg cholesterol; 470 mg sodium. EXCHANGES: 1 grain (starch); 1½ fat.

SERVING IDEA: Top the griddle cakes with warm brown rice syrup.

Oatmeal Breakfast Cake

Make ahead and reheat for a breakfast treat or between-meals snack.

MAKES 6 SERVINGS   PREPARATION TIME: 1 HOUR 10 MINUTES

Olive oil spray
2 cups old-fashioned rolled oats
¼ cup xylitol
⅓ cup chopped dried apricots
¾ teaspoon ground cinnamon
2½ cups nonfat milk
3 egg whites or ⅓ cup Egg Beaters or other egg white product
¾ tablespoon hazelnut oil or almond oil
¾ tablespoon vanilla extract

Preheat the oven to 350 degrees F. Spray an 8-by-8-inch baking dish with olive oil spray.

In a large mixing bowl, stir oats, xylitol, apricots, and cinnamon together until mixed well. Add milk, egg whites, oil, and vanilla and stir well until ingredients are blended.

Pour into the prepared baking dish. Bake 45 to 50 minutes, until just set.

PER SERVING: 205 calories; 4 g fat (15.0% calories from fat); 10 g protein; 36 g carbohydrate; 4 g dietary fiber; 2 mg cholesterol; 82 mg sodium. EXCHANGES: 1 grain (starch); ½ fruit; ½ nonfat milk; ½ fat.

Note
The beta-glucan and other soluble fiber in oats lower blood sugar and cholesterol levels, increase satiety, and may help promote weight loss.

Oat Bran–Apricot Muffins

Full of cholesterol-lowering oat bran.

MAKES 12 MUFFINS   PREPARATION TIME: 40 MINUTES

Olive oil spray
- ¾ cup orange juice or apple juice
- ¾ cup nonfat plain yogurt
- 2 egg whites or ¼ cup Egg Beaters or other egg white product
- 2 tablespoons brown rice syrup or honey
- 1½ cups old-fashioned rolled oats
- 1 cup oat bran
- 1 teaspoon baking soda
- ½ cup finely chopped dried apricots

Preheat the oven to 350 degrees F. Spray a 12-cup muffin tin with olive oil spray.

Combine juice, yogurt, egg whites, and syrup in a medium bowl and stir with a whisk until blended.

Combine rolled oats, oat bran, and baking soda in another bowl and stir until blended.

Fold dry ingredients into liquid ingredients, along with apricots, and stir until moistened. Spoon into muffin cups.

Bake for 15 to 20 minutes, until lightly browned. Let sit in muffin cups for about 5 minutes before removing.

PER SERVING: 102 calories; 1 g fat (9.6% calories from fat); 5 g protein; 22 g carbohydrate; 3 g dietary fiber; trace cholesterol; 130 mg sodium. EXCHANGES: 1 grain (starch); ½ fruit.

Note
When a recipe calls for dried fruit of any kind, use low-glycemic dried apricots.

Cinnamon-Applesauce Toast

Sure to please your kids—or the kid in you.

MAKES 4 SERVINGS   PREPARATION TIME: 10 MINUTES

  4   *slices sprouted-grain bread*
  1   *cup unsweetened applesauce*
1½   *tablespoons xylitol, or to taste*
 ½   *teaspoon ground cinnamon, or to taste*

Preheat the broiler or a toaster oven.

Toast one side of bread slices, placing about 3 inches below heating element for 1 to 3 minutes.

Meanwhile, mix applesauce, xylitol, and cinnamon together in a small bowl. Spread over untoasted side of bread slices.

Return bread to the toaster oven or broiler and cook 2 to 3 minutes, until applesauce is bubbly and edges of toast are brown.

PER SERVING: 118 calories; 1 g fat (3.8% calories from fat); 4 g protein; 27 g carbohydrate; 4 g dietary fiber; 0 mg cholesterol; 76 mg sodium. EXCHANGES: 1 grain (starch); ½ lean meat; ½ fruit.

Note

The dense texture of sprouted-grain bread works exceptionally well in this recipe. If you prefer your bread softer, skip the first step and toast it only on one side after you've added the applesauce.

Cheese "Danish"

Not exactly a cheese Danish, but a healthful alternative.

MAKES 4 SERVINGS   PREPARATION TIME: 10 MINUTES

1 cup low-fat cottage cheese
2 tablespoons xylitol or 5 to 6 drops stevia, to taste
½ teaspoon ground cinnamon (optional)
½ cup peach slices in juice (no added sugar), drained
4 slices sprouted-grain bread

Preheat the broiler or a toaster oven to high.

Mix cottage cheese, xylitol (or stevia), and cinnamon together in a small bowl.

Cut peaches into thin slices.

Toast one side of bread slices, placing about 3 inches from heating element and cooking for 1 to 3 minutes.

Spread ¼ cup cottage cheese mixture on untoasted side of each slice of toast. Arrange peach slices on cottage cheese.

Return to broiler or toaster oven and cook 2 to 3 minutes, until heated through.

PER SERVING: 150 calories; 1 g fat (6.1% calories from fat); 11 g protein; 26 g carbohydrate; 3 g dietary fiber; 2 mg cholesterol; 306 mg sodium. EXCHANGES: 1 grain (starch); 1½ lean meat.

SERVING IDEA: Replace peaches with 1 tablespoon of unsweetened applesauce or other fruit.

Blueberry Muffins

Bursting with the flavor and health benefits of blueberries.

MAKES 12 MUFFINS   PREPARATION TIME: 30 MINUTES

   Olive oil spray
 2 cups oat bran
 ¼ cup xylitol
 2 teaspoons baking powder
 ¼ teaspoon baking soda
 4 egg whites or ½ cup Egg Beaters or other egg white product
 ½ cup orange juice
 ½ cup nonfat plain yogurt
 2 tablespoons hazelnut oil or almond oil
 ¾ cup fresh or frozen blueberries (do not thaw)

Preheat the oven to 350 degrees F. Spray a 12-cup muffin tin with olive oil spray.

In a large bowl, mix oat bran, xylitol, baking powder, and baking soda and stir until well blended.

In a medium bowl, mix egg whites, orange juice, yogurt, and oil with a wire whisk until smooth.

Fold liquid mixture into oat bran mixture and stir until moistened. Gently fold in blueberries.

Fill muffin cups three-fourths full. Bake for 16 minutes, until lightly browned. To test for doneness, stick a toothpick into center of muffin. It should come out clean. Cool for 5 minutes for easier removal from muffin cups.

PER SERVING: 89 calories; 3 g fat (25.8% calories from fat); 5 g protein; 18 g carbohydrate; 3 g dietary fiber; trace cholesterol; 134 mg sodium. EXCHANGES: ½ grain (starch); ½ fat.

SERVING IDEAS: These muffins are best served warm. Store cooled muffins in a tightly sealed bag in the refrigerator. They also make a good snack.

Note
Because these muffins contain no flour, they are dense, moist, and somewhat crumbly. On the plus side, they won't mess with your blood sugar as regular muffins do.

Apricot-Oat Granola Bars

A nutrient-dense breakfast you can eat on the run.

MAKES 12 BARS   PREPARATION TIME: 30 MINUTES

Olive oil spray
½ cup brown rice syrup
⅓ cup whole wheat flour
1 tablespoon hazelnut oil or almond oil
2 teaspoons vanilla extract
2 cups old-fashioned rolled oats
1 cup raw sunflower seeds
½ cup oat bran
½ cup finely chopped dried apricots

Preheat the oven to 350 degrees F. Spray an 8-by-8-inch baking dish with olive oil spray.

Combine brown rice syrup, flour, and hazelnut oil in a small saucepan over medium heat. Cook until hot and thin, but not quite boiling, 2 to 3 minutes. Remove from the heat and stir in vanilla.

Combine oats, sunflower seeds, oat bran, and dried apricots in a large bowl and mix well. Pour syrup over oat mixture and stir well to evenly coat.

Using your hands, press into the prepared baking dish. (This will be sticky. To make it easier and less messy, put your hand in a plastic bag, spray a little oil on the bag, and press.) Bars will be ½ to ¾ inch thick.

Bake for 10 to 15 minutes, until bottom is brown. Cool 10 minutes, then cut into bars.

PER SERVING: 221 calories; 8 g fat (30.7% calories from fat); 7 g protein; 35 g carbohydrate; 4 g dietary fiber; 0 mg cholesterol; 17 mg sodium. EXCHANGES: 1 grain (starch); ½ lean meat; 1½ fat.

SERVING IDEA: These are also good as a between-meal snack.

Note

Don't be put off by the fairly high fat and carbohydrate content in these bars. Most of the fat is healthful poly- and monounsaturated fat, and the carbohydrates in oats and bran do not cause spikes in blood sugar.

Applesauce Muffins

These cinnamon-scented muffins make a good snack.

MAKES 12 MUFFINS   PREPARATION TIME: 35 MINUTES

   1 *cup oat bran*
   1 *cup whole wheat flour*
  ½ *cup xylitol*
  ½ *cup chopped dried apricots*
  ¼ *cup chopped pecans or other nuts*
 1⅓ *teaspoons baking powder*
 1⅓ *teaspoons baking soda*
  ½ *teaspoon ground cinnamon*
  ⅓ *teaspoon salt or salt substitute*
   3 *egg whites or ⅓ cup Egg Beaters or other egg white product*
  ⅔ *cup unsweetened applesauce, chilled*
 2½ *tablespoons hazelnut oil or almond oil*
       Olive oil spray

In a large mixing bowl, mix oat bran, flour, xylitol, apricots, pecans, baking powder, baking soda, cinnamon, and salt. Add egg whites, applesauce, and hazelnut oil. Stir until well blended.

Preheat the oven to 400 degrees F. Spray a 12-cup muffin tin with olive oil spray. Fill the cups three-fourths full and let stand for 10 minutes.

Bake for 12 to 15 minutes, until centers spring back when lightly touched.

PER SERVING: 141 calories; 5 g fat (27.0% calories from fat); 4 g protein; 27 g carbohydrate; 3 g dietary fiber; 0 mg cholesterol; 269 mg sodium. EXCHANGES: 1 grain (starch); ½ fruit; 1 fat.

Note

Hazelnut oil has even more healthy monounsaturated fats than olive oil. Almond and avocado oils are other milder-tasting monos.

Appetizers

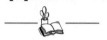

Appetizers are meant to be served in small portions before a meal to "stimulate the appetite." For most of us, however, multicourse meals are the exception rather than the rule. Nevertheless, it's nice to have a few appetizers up your sleeve to serve at special meals and parties. Unfortunately, many hors d'oeuvres, canapés, dips, and other finger foods are a minefield of saturated fats and refined carbs. Not these appetizers. They are all designed to keep your blood sugar on an even keel and provide you with a wealth of vitamins, minerals, healthy fats, and protective phytonutrients.

The selection of appetizers in this chapter ranges from the exotic (Black Olive Tapenade, page 66) to the elegant (Classic Shrimp Cocktail, page 73) to the informal (Brandon's Bean Dip, page 61). Some of them also make a good main course: Chicken Satay with Thai Peanut Sauce (page 74), for example. Others, such as Creamy Smoked Salmon (page 72), are terrific sandwich spreads. And virtually all of these appetizers are perfect between-meal snacks.

Guacamole

A cool, creamy dip or topping for Mexican food.

2 medium ripe avocados
3 tablespoons lime juice or lemon juice
1 tablespoon Mary's Fresh Salsa (page 283) or Quick and Easy
  Salsa (page 284) or store-bought salsa
¼ teaspoon salt or salt substitute
1 clove garlic, peeled and minced
3 tablespoons canned chopped mild green chiles (optional)
1 small tomato, chopped
¼ cup chopped onion
2 tablespoons freshly chopped cilantro (optional)

In a medium bowl, mash avocados with a fork until smooth. Add lime juice, salsa, salt, garlic, and chiles and stir until well blended. Gently stir in tomato, onion, and cilantro.

PER SERVING (includes salsa): 122 calories; 10 g fat (69.9% calories from fat); 2 g protein; 8 g carbohydrate; 2 g dietary fiber; 0 mg cholesterol; 124 mg sodium. EXCHANGES: ½ vegetable; ½ fruit; 2 fat.

SERVING IDEA: Use this as a dip, or serve a spoonful with burritos, fajitas, tacos, and other Mexican dishes.

Note

Avocados are high in fat, but it's mostly healthful monounsaturated fat. They do contain a lot of calories, so eat in moderation.

Tapas Trio

Colorful, quick, trendy munchies from Spain.

MAKES 4 SERVINGS (½ CUP EACH)   PREPARATION TIME: 30 MINUTES

1   *cup mushrooms*
1   *teaspoon extra-virgin olive oil*
1   *teaspoon balsamic vinegar or lemon juice*
¼   *teaspoon Low-Sodium Seasoned Salt (page 297)
    or salt substitute*
½   *clove garlic, peeled and minced*
¼   *cup green olives*
¼   *cup ripe olives (preferably kalamata)*
1   *(4-ounce) tin sardines in tomato sauce or mustard, drained*
3   *teaspoons freshly chopped parsley, for garnish*

Clean mushrooms and cut in half, if small, or quarters, if large.

Combine olive oil, vinegar, seasoned salt, and garlic in a small serving bowl. Stir, then add mushrooms and mix until evenly coated. Allow to marinate at room temperature for 15 to 30 minutes. (If longer, cover and place in refrigerator.)

Drain green and ripe olives and place in a small serving bowl.

Drain sardines and place in a small serving bowl.

Garnish each dish with 1 teaspoon parsley and serve.

PER SERVING: 86 calories; 6 g fat (66.2% calories from fat); 5 g protein; 2 g carbohydrate; 1 g dietary fiber; 17 mg cholesterol; 352 mg sodium. EXCHANGES: ½ lean meat; 1 fat.

SERVING IDEA: You can add marinated zucchini, artichoke hearts, roasted red peppers, small pieces of cooked, spiced chicken . . . the possibilities are limitless. Serve in small bowls, pour the wine, and dig in!

Note

Tapas are Spain's version of appetizers and a standard in bars, where small portions of an often dizzying array of tapas are served.

Spicy Hummus

A spicy version of a classic dip.

MAKES 6 SERVINGS (1½ CUPS)   PREPARATION TIME: 10 MINUTES

1   *(15½-ounce) can garbanzo beans, rinsed and drained, or*
    1½ cups cooked garbanzos
3   *tablespoons water*
¼   *cup tahini (see Note)*
3   *teaspoons extra-virgin olive oil*
2   *tablespoons lemon juice*
2   *cloves garlic, peeled and chopped*
¼   *teaspoon ground cumin*
½   *teaspoon plus dash cayenne pepper, or to taste*
¼   *teaspoon salt or salt substitute*
3   *parsley sprigs, for garnish*

Combine beans, water, tahini, 2 teaspoons olive oil, lemon juice, garlic, cumin, ½ teaspoon cayenne pepper, and salt in a food processor or blender and process until smooth, adding a little more water if needed to achieve a soft, creamy consistency.

Transfer to a serving dish. Top with remaining teaspoon of olive oil and dash of cayenne pepper. Garnish with parsley sprigs.

PER SERVING: 101 calories; 5 g fat (46.8% calories from fat); 3 g protein; 11 g carbohydrate; 2 g dietary fiber; 0 mg cholesterol; 215 mg sodium. EXCHANGES: ½ grain (starch); 1 fat.

SERVING IDEA: Serve this with triangles of whole-grain pita bread. (Limit bread to 1 slice per serving.)

Note
Tahini is sesame seed butter. Look for it in the ethnic section of your supermarket.

Grecian Mushrooms

Stuffed with spinach and feta cheese.

MAKES 4 SERVINGS (16 MUSHROOMS)   PREPARATION TIME: 45 MINUTES

Olive oil spray
1   (10-ounce) package frozen spinach, defrosted and drained
16 medium fresh mushrooms
½   cup feta cheese
1   tablespoon grated Parmesan cheese
¼   teaspoon freshly ground black pepper

Preheat the oven to 375 degrees F. Spray a shallow 8-by-8-inch baking dish with olive oil spray.

Squeeze excess moisture out of spinach.

Clean mushrooms, remove stems and discard, or save for another use.

In a medium bowl, mix spinach and feta cheese until blended.

Stuff mushroom caps with spinach mixture, making a mound of spinach on top of each mushroom. Sprinkle each with a pinch of Parmesan cheese and black pepper.

Place in the baking dish and bake for 30 minutes, or until tender.

PER SERVING: 90 calories; 5 g fat (44.3% calories from fat); 7 g protein; 7 g carbohydrate; 3 g dietary fiber; 18 mg cholesterol; 288 mg sodium. EXCHANGES: ½ lean meat; 1½ vegetable; ½ fat.

SERVING IDEA: You may have some spinach-feta mixture left over. Save it for a dip. When ready to serve, place it in a small glass bowl, and heat in the microwave for 2 minutes or until hot and bubbly. Serve with whole wheat pita triangles.

(continued)

Grecian Mushrooms *(continued)*

Note

Cheese is not off limits in a healthy diet. Eat it in small quantities and go for strong-flavored cheese like feta: a little goes a long way.

Brandon's Bean Dip

A quick and easy snack created by one of our college boys.

MAKES 6 SERVINGS (2 CUPS)   PREPARATION TIME: 10 MINUTES

1 *can nonfat refried beans or 1½ cups cooked pinto beans*
2 *tablespoons Mary's Fresh Salsa (page 283) or Quick and Easy Salsa (page 284) or store-bought salsa, or to taste*
½ *cup fat-free sour cream*
½ *cup grated sharp Cheddar cheese*
2 *tablespoons freshly chopped cilantro, for garnish (optional)*

Mix all ingredients except for cilantro and stir until well blended. (If you're using whole beans, mash with a fork or process in a blender or food processor.)

Place in a covered microwave-proof dish and heat for about 2 minutes, stirring occasionally, until hot and bubbly (or heat in a small saucepan for 3 to 5 minutes). Garnish with cilantro.

PER SERVING (includes salsa): 96 calories; 3 g fat (29% calories from fat); 6 g protein; 11 g carbohydrate; 1 g dietary fiber; 12 mg cholesterol; 310 mg sodium. EXCHANGES: ½ lean meat; ½ fat; ½ other carbohydrates.

SERVING IDEAS: Serve this with fat-free chips, carrots, celery, and green peppers. (Go easy on the chips.) You can also turn this into a main dish by spooning it into a warm tortilla and topping it with chopped tomatoes, onions, lettuce, and salsa.

Note
Beans are an excellent source of soluble fiber, which lowers blood sugar in people with diabetes. Recent studies show that eating 50 grams of fiber a day lowers blood sugar by 10 percent.

Emerald Dip

Rich and creamy.

MAKES 12 SERVINGS (3 CUPS)   PREPARATION TIME: 4 HOURS 10 MINUTES

1   (10-ounce) package frozen chopped spinach
1   cup low-fat mayonnaise
1   cup low-fat sour cream
½   cup freshly chopped parsley
½   cup chopped green onions
1   clove garlic, peeled and minced
½   teaspoon Low-Sodium Seasoned Salt (page 297) or salt substitute
¼   teaspoon freshly ground black pepper

Thaw spinach, drain, and squeeze moisture out until dry.

Combine spinach with remaining ingredients in a medium bowl and mix well.

Cover and refrigerate at least 2 hours, or overnight.

Stir before serving, and add 1 to 2 tablespoons of milk to thin, if desired.

PER SERVING: 103 calories; 10 g fat (80.7% calories from fat); 1 g protein; 4 g carbohydrate; 1 g dietary fiber; 15 mg cholesterol; 181 mg sodium. EXCHANGES: ½ vegetable; 2 fat.

SERVING IDEAS: Serve with raw vegetables, such as carrot and celery sticks, green or red pepper slices, broccoli and cauliflower florets, and cherry tomatoes. One small can of cooked clams, drained and chopped, makes a nice addition.

Cherry Tomato Surprises

Particularly good during the summer, when tomatoes are at their best.

MAKES 6 SERVINGS   PREPARATION TIME: 20 MINUTES

1 *pound (about 30) cherry tomatoes*
⅓ *cup fat-free cream cheese*
¼ *cup freshly chopped parsley*
¼ *teaspoon garlic powder*
1 *tablespoon pitted and chopped black olives*
1 *tablespoon freshly grated Parmesan cheese*
¼ *teaspoon freshly ground black pepper*

Rinse tomatoes and cut top quarter off each tomato. Remove seeds and insides. Chop 1 tablespoon of tomatoes (from top quarters) and set aside; discard the rest, leaving only tomato shells.

Combine remaining ingredients. Fill tomatoes with mixture, then refrigerate and cover until ready to serve. Filling may be made ahead of time, but fill tomatoes no more than 2 hours before serving.

PER SERVING: 33 calories; 1 g fat (20.0% calories from fat); 3 g protein; 4 g carbohydrate; 1 g dietary fiber; 2 mg cholesterol; 103 mg sodium. EXCHANGES: ½ lean meat; ½ vegetable.

Note
Tomatoes are one of nature's richest sources of lycopene. This red pigment is a potent antioxidant that protects against cancer and heart disease.

Cheesy Roll-Ups
Fun finger food.

MAKES 6 SERVINGS   PREPARATION TIME: 3 HOURS 15 MINUTES

2 tablespoons minced ripe olives
¼ cup minced red bell pepper
¼ cup minced green onions
½ cup low-fat sour cream
½ cup grated sharp Cheddar cheese
1 tablespoon freshly chopped parsley
3 whole wheat tortillas

In a medium mixing bowl, combine olives, red pepper, onions, sour cream, cheese, and parsley.

Divide among tortillas and spread evenly over one side of each, making sure cheese mixture extends to edges of tortillas. Roll up tortillas tightly.

Wrap individual tortillas in plastic wrap and refrigerate for at least 3 hours or overnight.

Before serving, cut each tortilla into 1-inch slices.

PER SERVING: 105 calories; 5 g fat (36.1% calories from fat); 5 g protein; 13 g carbohydrate; trace dietary fiber; 14 mg cholesterol; 193 mg sodium. EXCHANGES: 1 grain (starch); ½ lean meat; ½ fat; other carbohydrates.

Note
You can roll up most any filling in tortillas: refried beans, cheese, and salsa; smoked salmon and cream cheese; hummus and olives. . . . Be creative!

Buttery Roasted Garlic

Surprisingly mellow and buttery smooth.

MAKES 2 SERVINGS PREPARATION TIME: 45 MINUTES

1 *head garlic*
2 *teaspoons extra-virgin olive oil*
¼ *teaspoon Low-Sodium Seasoned Salt (page 297) or salt substitute*
2 *slices pumpernickel bread*

Preheat the oven to 350 degrees F.

Loosen garlic cloves, but do not remove from head. Pour olive oil over garlic and sprinkle with seasoned salt. Place in a small, covered baking dish or wrap in aluminum foil and roast until soft, 30 to 45 minutes (depending on size of garlic).

Meanwhile, toast pumpernickel bread and cut into small triangles.

Serve garlic with bread (see Serving Ideas).

PER SERVING: 123 calories; 6 g fat (39.9% calories from fat); 3 g protein; 16 g carbohydrate; 2 g dietary fiber; 0 mg cholesterol; 386 mg sodium. EXCHANGES: 1 grain (starch); 1 fat.

SERVING IDEAS: Place the whole garlic on a plate with toast triangles. Diners remove individual cloves, squeeze garlic from the peels (it will be soft and buttery), and spread it on toast. You may also remove all the garlic from the cloves, mash with a fork, and serve as a spread.

Note
For a variation, tuck a sprig of rosemary or another favorite herb into the baking dish or foil before cooking.

Black Olive Tapenade

A Mediterranean classic.

MAKES 12 SERVINGS (2 CUPS)   PREPARATION TIME: 10 MINUTES

2 *cups ripe olives (preferably kalamata)*
¼ *cup capers (optional)*
1 *(2-ounce) can anchovy fillets, rinsed, or ¼ cup sardines, drained*
1 *clove garlic, peeled and minced*
3 *tablespoons lemon juice*
1 *teaspoon freshly chopped thyme or ¼ teaspoon dried thyme*
1 *teaspoon freshly chopped rosemary or ¼ teaspoon dried rosemary*
3 *tablespoons extra-virgin olive oil*

Combine olives, capers, anchovies, garlic, lemon juice, thyme, and rosemary in a food processor or blender and process until smooth. Slowly add olive oil and process until you have a smooth paste.

PER SERVING: 67 calories; 6 g fat (80.5% calories from fat); 2 g protein; 2 g carbohydrate; 1 g dietary fiber; 4 mg cholesterol; 396 mg sodium. EXCHANGE: 1 fat.

SERVING IDEAS: Serve tapenade as a dip for raw or roasted vegetables or on sprouted-grain toast triangles. This intensely flavored delicacy may also be spread on skinless chicken breasts, fish fillets, or vegetables before grilling, broiling, or roasting. In addition, it can be tossed with pasta and lightly sautéed vegetables (chopped zucchini, onions, tomatoes).

Baba Ganoush

A deliciously different Middle Eastern dip made with eggplant.

MAKES 6 SERVINGS (2 CUPS)   PREPARATION TIME: 2 HOURS 30 MINUTES

1   *large or 2 medium eggplants*
¼   *cup tahini (see Note, page 58)*
2   *cloves garlic, peeled and minced*
2   *tablespoons lemon juice*
½   *teaspoon salt or salt substitute*
2   *tablespoons freshly chopped parsley*

Preheat the oven to 400 degrees F.

Prick skin of eggplant with a fork, place in a baking dish, and bake for 40 to 50 minutes, depending on size, until soft and wrinkled.

Let eggplant cool for 15 to 20 minutes, until you can handle it; cutting it open helps it cool faster. Then cut in half and scrape "meat" out of skin.

Place eggplant, tahini, garlic, lemon juice, and salt in a medium bowl and mash with a fork until blended. (You may also use a food processor or blender.)

Transfer to a serving bowl and sprinkle with parsley. Cover and chill at least 1 hour before serving.

PER SERVING: 83 calories; 6 g fat (54.9% calories from fat); 3 g protein; 8 g carbohydrate; 3 g dietary fiber; 0 mg cholesterol; 192 mg sodium. EXCHANGES: 1 vegetable; 1 fat.

SERVING IDEAS: Serve this with whole-grain pita bread, cut into triangles.

Antipasto Platter

An easy, traditional first course to an Italian dinner.

MAKES 4 SERVINGS   PREPARATION TIME: 20 MINUTES

  4 *large romaine leaves*
  ¾ *cup marinated artichoke hearts, rinsed, drained, and halved*
  ½ *cup roasted red peppers*
  ½ *cup pepperoncini peppers, whole, drained*
  2 *medium tomatoes, cut into ½-inch wedges*
  ½ *medium green bell pepper, thinly sliced*
  ½ *cup black olives (preferably kalamata)*
  2 *ounces provolone cheese slices, rolled up, cigar style*
  2 *ounces turkey salami slices*

Place romaine leaves on a large platter. Arrange other ingredients attractively in groups on romaine.

PER SERVING: 163 calories; 10 g fat (53.6% calories from fat); 9 g protein; 11 g carbohydrate; 4 g dietary fiber; 21 mg cholesterol; 565 mg sodium. EXCHANGES: ½ lean meat; 1½ vegetable; 1½ fat.

SERVING IDEA: Diners help themselves to their favorites on the Antipasto Platter.

Note
You'll find roasted red peppers, pepperoncinis, and other Italian delicacies in the gourmet section of your grocery store. You can make any number of variations of antipasto by using green olives, other types of peppers, canned sardines or anchovies, green onions, and other raw vegetables.

Baja Shrimp

A nice change from shrimp cocktail.

MAKES 8 SERVINGS   PREPARATION TIME: 2 HOURS 10 MINUTES

1 *pound (30 to 35) medium shrimp*
2 *cloves garlic, peeled and minced*
½ *cup lime juice*
½ *teaspoon grated lime peel*
1 *tablespoon extra-virgin olive oil*
¼ *cup chopped green onion*
¼ *cup freshly chopped cilantro*
½ *cup Anaheim chiles (see Note)*
1 *tablespoon jalapeño chiles (canned or fresh), seeds removed (optional) (see Note)*
½ *teaspoon salt or salt substitute*
¼ *teaspoon freshly ground black pepper*
   Whole cilantro leaves, for garnish

Prepare shrimp. If frozen and cooked, simply thaw under cold running water. If raw, cook by bringing 3 cups of water to a boil, adding shrimp, and cooking for 2 to 3 minutes, until shrimp turn pink. Rinse, drain, and cool. Peel, including tails, and remove veins.

Combine remaining ingredients except cilantro garnish in a medium bowl. Add cooked shrimp, stir well, and marinate in the refrigerator for 2 to 3 hours, stirring occasionally.

Pour off marinade and garnish with cilantro leaves.

PER SERVING: 88 calories; 3 g fat (27.9% calories from fat); 12 g protein; 4 g carbohydrate; trace dietary fiber; 86 mg cholesterol; 221 mg sodium. EXCHANGES: 1½ lean meat; ½ vegetable; ½ fat.

(continued)

Baja Shrimp *(continued)*

Note

Anaheim chiles are long, slender peppers that are mildly to moderately hot. If you can't find them, use canned green chiles. Add fiery hot jalapeños at your own discretion.

Catalina Crab Dip
Delicious with raw vegetables.

MAKES 6 SERVINGS (1½ CUPS)   PREPARATION TIME: 15 MINUTES

8 ounces low-fat cream cheese, softened
4 ounces crabmeat or surimi (see Note), coarsely chopped
1 tablespoon skim milk
1 teaspoon lemon juice
¼ cup finely chopped green onions
1 small clove garlic peeled and minced
¼ teaspoon Low-Sodium Seasoned Salt (page 297) or salt substitute
1 tomato, chopped
2 tablespoons freshly chopped parsley or cilantro

Mix cream cheese, crabmeat, milk, lemon juice, green onions, garlic, and salt thoroughly with a fork.

Spread over the bottom of a 6- to 8-inch plate.

Cover and refrigerate until ready to serve. Just before serving top with tomato and sprinkle with parsley or cilantro.

PER SERVING: 114 calories; 7 g fat (55.3% calories from fat); 8 g protein; 4 g carbohydrate; trace dietary fiber; 38 mg cholesterol; 388 mg sodium. EXCHANGES: 1 lean meat; ½ vegetable; 1 fat.

SERVING IDEA: Serve this with raw vegetables.

Note
Surimi, imitation seafood, is made from mild-flavored fish such as Alaskan pollock blended with concentrates from shellfish. It's high in protein, low in fat (although a bit salty), and much less expensive than crab and shrimp.

Creamy Smoked Salmon

A great way to stretch the wonderful flavor of smoked salmon.

MAKES 6 SERVINGS (1½ CUPS)   PREPARATION TIME: 10 MINUTES

 4 *ounces smoked salmon*
 8 *ounces nonfat cream cheese, softened*
 2 *tablespoons fat-free mayonnaise*
 2 *tablespoons minced green onion*
 ½ *teaspoon lemon juice*
 ¼ *teaspoon Worcestershire sauce*

Blend all ingredients well with a fork.

Shape into a log, or place in a serving dish. Keeps in refrigerator for a week.

PER SERVING: 114 calories; 7 g fat (59.6% calories from fat); 7 g protein; 4 g carbohydrate; trace dietary fiber; 26 mg cholesterol; 477 mg sodium. EXCHANGES: 1 lean meat; 1 fat.

SERVING IDEAS: Serve this with toasted 100 percent rye or sprouted-grain bread, cut into triangles. (You should go easy on crackers, since foods made with flour tend to raise blood sugar levels.) This also makes a good sandwich filling.

Note

A 7-ounce can of water-packed tuna, well drained, may be substituted for the smoked salmon.

Classic Shrimp Cocktail

An appetizer you can't go wrong with.

MAKES 6 SERVINGS   PREPARATION TIME: 20 MINUTES

1   *pound (20 to 25) large shrimp*
½   *cup ketchup*
¼   *teaspoon horseradish, or to taste*
½   *teaspoon lemon juice*
4   *romaine leaves*
1   *lemon, cut into eighths*

Prepare shrimp. If frozen, simply thaw under cold running water. If raw, cook by bringing 3 cups of water to a boil, adding shrimp, and cooking for 2 or 3 minutes, until shrimp turn pink. Rinse, drain, and cool. Peel, leaving tails intact, and devein.

Make Cocktail Sauce by combining ketchup, horseradish, and lemon juice in a small bowl and mixing well. Refrigerate.

Cover the bottom of a large plate with romaine leaves. Place the bowl of Cocktail Sauce in the center of the plate. Arrange shrimp in a circular pattern on romaine leaves. Garnish with lemon wedges and serve.

PER SERVING: 104 calories; 1 g fat (11.8% calories from fat); 16 g protein; 7 g carbohydrate; trace dietary fiber; 115 mg cholesterol; 350 mg sodium. EXCHANGES: 2 lean meat; ½ other carbohydrates.

SERVING IDEA: Another serving idea is to place cocktail sauce in martini glasses and drape the shrimp over the edges of the glasses, tails on the outside.

Chicken Satay with Thai Peanut Sauce

Marinated skewered chicken—a Southeast Asian standard.

MAKES 8 SERVINGS   PREPARATION TIME: 2 HOURS 20 MINUTES

- 1 pound skinless, boneless chicken breast
- 2 cloves garlic, peeled and minced
- 1 tablespoon extra-virgin olive oil
- 1 tablespoon low-sodium soy sauce
- 1 tablespoon lemon juice
- ½ teaspoon curry powder
- 16 (6-inch) bamboo skewers
- 8 romaine leaves
- ¾ cup Thai Peanut Sauce (page 292)

Cut chicken breast lengthwise into long, thin slices, approximately 1 by 4 by ¼ inches. (Put chicken in freezer for 20 minutes for easier slicing.)

Mix garlic, olive oil, soy sauce, lemon juice, and curry powder in a small bowl, then transfer marinade to a plastic bag along with chicken. Squeeze the air out, seal, and refrigerate for at least 2 hours, turning the bag every half hour or so.

Meanwhile, soak the bamboo skewers in water for at least 30 minutes.

Thread chicken slices onto skewers, working the skewer in and out along the chicken. Baste both sides with marinade.

Preheat the broiler (or a grill or barbecue) to high, then place the skewers on the broiler plate or grill and cook for 2 to 3 minutes on each side, until golden brown. (Watch carefully to prevent burning.)

Serve the Chicken Satay on romaine leaves. Dip in the peanut sauce.

PER SERVING (includes Thai Peanut Sauce): 151 calories; 8 g fat (45% calories from fat); 16 g protein; 5 g carbohydrate; 1 g dietary fiber; 33 mg cholesterol; 213 mg sodium. EXCHANGES: 2 lean meat; 1½ fat.

SERVING IDEAS: Chicken Satay can also be served as a main dish. Allow 4 ounces of chicken per main dish serving and use longer, 10- to 12-inch skewers if desired. Pair it with Thai Noodles (page 272) and Stir-Fried Asparagus (page 255).

Note
Trimmed lean beef or cleaned shrimp may be used in place of chicken.

Beverages

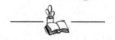

Purified water is the beverage of choice, and, as you know, you should drink a minimum of eight glasses of water daily. Yet sometimes you have the urge for something different to drink, and if you're trying to stay on the straight and narrow, your selections may seem somewhat limited. The safety of artificial sweeteners is questionable. Soft drinks ("liquid sugar") contain an average of ten teaspoons of high-fructose corn syrup. Fruit "drinks," despite their name, are little more than sugar water with added fruit flavoring. Even pure fruit juices are a concentrated source of sugar and calories.

Broaden your horizons with the beverages in this chapter. The fruit-based recipes use diluted juices or whole fruit, which have a less drastic impact on blood sugar. The tea and coffee drinks are extraordinary versions of ordinary beverages, and we've even provided a couple of alcoholic drinks. Most diabetics, unless their blood sugar is poorly controlled, can drink a little alcohol. Alcohol not only protects against heart disease but modest amounts actually lower blood sugar by improving the cells' sensitivity to insulin.

That said, a few words of caution are in order. First, don't drink alcohol without food—it could cause your blood sugar to go too low. Second, drink moderately: no more than two drinks a day for men and one for women, who metabolize alcohol more slowly than men. Any more than that can have adverse consequences. Third, if you have liver disease or other health conditions, or if you're taking medications that interact with alcohol, avoid it. Finally, alcohol has a tremendous potential for abuse. If you are a person who cannot handle alcohol, don't use its health benefits as an excuse to drink.

Citrus Spritzer
Tart and delicious.

2   cups lemon-flavored sparkling water
1   cup orange juice
½   cup lemon juice
½   cup lime juice
10 drops stevia or ⅓ cup xylitol, to taste

Combine all ingredients in a large pitcher. Stir well and chill. Serve over ice.

PER SERVING: 44 calories; trace fat (2.7% calories from fat); 1 g protein; 12 g carbohydrate; trace dietary fiber; 0 mg cholesterol; 1 mg sodium. EXCHANGE: 1 fruit.

Note
If you like to drink juice but don't like what it does to your blood sugar, dilute it with sparkling water.

Orange Slush

Smooth and icy cold—with the RDA of vitamin C.

MAKES 4 SERVINGS (4 CUPS)   PREPARATION TIME: 5 MINUTES

2 *oranges, peeled and quartered*
6 *tablespoons frozen concentrate orange juice*
1 *tablespoon lemon juice*
2 *cups ice*
1 *cup water*

Place all ingredients in a blender. Process until smooth and thick.

PER SERVING: 74 calories; trace fat (1.5% calories from fat); 1 g protein; 18 g carbohydrate; 2 g dietary fiber; 0 mg cholesterol; 6 mg sodium. EXCHANGE: 1 fruit.

Note
Substitute tangerines for a different taste.

Peach Smoothie

A creamy, high-protein drink that makes a healthy snack.

MAKES 2 SERVINGS (3 CUPS)   PREPARATION TIME: 5 MINUTES

⅓ *cup nonfat plain yogurt*
1 *cup water*
1 *scoop protein powder*
1½ *cups frozen peach slices*
½ *cup ice cubes*
8 *drops stevia or 1 to 2 tablespoons xylitol, to taste*

Combine yogurt, water, and protein powder in a blender. With the blender running, add peach slices, a few at a time, through opening in the lid, blending until smooth. Add ice cubes, 1 at a time, and blend until thick and smooth. Add stevia, process, and taste. Add more stevia, 1 drop at a time, until desired sweetness is achieved. (Or add xylitol, 1 tablespoon at a time.)

PER SERVING: 126 calories; 1 g fat (6.4% calories from fat); 12 g protein; 18 g carbohydrate; 3 g dietary fiber; 16 mg cholesterol; 54 mg sodium. EXCHANGES: 1½ lean meat; 1 fruit; ½ nonfat milk.

Note

Fresh or canned peaches (in juice or water, not syrup) may be substituted. Use 1 cup ice and ½ cup water, adding more water if needed to achieve desired consistency.

Sugar-Free Lemonade
Sweetened with stevia.

MAKES 4 SERVINGS   PREPARATION TIME: 5 MINUTES

4 *cups water*
⅔ *cup lemon juice*
15 to 20 drops stevia or ⅓ cup xylitol, to taste

Place water, lemon juice, and stevia (or xylitol) in a large pitcher and stir to dissolve. Serve chilled or over ice.

PER SERVING: 10 calories; 0 g fat (0.0% calories from fat); trace protein; 4 g carbohydrate; trace dietary fiber; 0 mg cholesterol; 8 mg sodium

Note

Most fresh or frozen lemonade is sweetened with high fructose corn syrup. Although fructose doesn't trigger a rapid rise in blood sugar, it has other adverse consequences for diabetics. It raises cholesterol levels, increases risk of heart disease, and combines with proteins to form compounds that are implicated in diabetic complications. Stevia, on the other hand, is completely safe and calorie free. Warning: Go easy on stevia. Add just a few drops of liquid or shakes of powdered stevia, taste, and add more, if needed. Some people find that stevia, especially if you overdo it, has an unpleasant aftertaste.

Virgin Strawberry Daiquiri

A nonalcoholic version of a favorite drink.

MAKES 2 SERVINGS   PREPARATION TIME: 5 MINUTES

¼ cup fresh lime juice
1 cup water
2 tablespoons xylitol
1¼ cups frozen strawberries (no sugar added)
¾ cup ice cubes

Combine lime juice, water, and xylitol in a blender. Add strawberries, 1 or 2 at a time, then ice cubes, 1 at a time, while blending. Process until smooth.

PER SERVING: 65 calories; trace fat (3.4% calories from fat); 1 g protein; 21 g carbohydrate; 2 g dietary fiber; 0 mg cholesterol; 7 mg sodium. EXCHANGE: ½ fruit.

SERVING IDEA: If you want to be really decadent, run a lime around the rims of daiquiri glasses, dip them in xylitol, and pour the daiquiris into the glasses.

Note

You can use any kind of fruit to make daiquiris—raspberries, blueberries, peaches, oranges, etc. The sweeter the fruit, the less sweetener you'll have to add. For a lower-carb version, substitute xylitol with 8 to 10 drops stevia (or to taste).

Mango Lassi

A traditional cool yogurt-fruit drink from India.

MAKES 4 SERVINGS   PREPARATION TIME: 10 MINUTES

1   *cup nonfat plain yogurt*
1   *cup ice cubes*
1   *cup mango (fresh, frozen, or canned and drained)*
½   *cup water*
3   *tablespoons xylitol or 8 to 10 drops stevia, to taste*
½   *teaspoon lemon juice*

Put all ingredients into a blender. Blend until smooth. Serve cold.

PER SERVING: 80 calories; trace fat (1.9% calories from fat); 3 g protein; 20 g carbohydrate; 1 g dietary fiber; 1 mg cholesterol; 47 mg sodium. EXCHANGES: ½ fruit; ½ nonfat milk.

Note
Lassi can also be made with oranges. Substitute 1 whole, peeled orange for the mango.

Virgin Bloody Mary

A tangy, refreshing potassium-rich drink.

MAKES 2 SERVINGS   PREPARATION TIME: 5 MINUTES

12 *ounces low-sodium V8 juice*
 2 *tablespoons lemon juice*
 1 *teaspoon Worcestershire sauce*
 2 *dashes Tabasco sauce, or to taste*
 2 *pinches freshly ground black pepper*
 2 *pinches celery salt*
   Ice cubes
 1 *stalk celery, trimmed and cut in half, for garnish*
 ½ *lime, cut into 2 wedges, for garnish*

Combine V8 juice, lemon juice, Worcestershire sauce, Tabasco sauce, pepper, and celery salt in a small pitcher. Stir to mix well. Pour into 2 glasses over ice cubes and garnish each with celery stick and lime wedge.

PER SERVING: 52 calories; trace fat (1.4% calories from fat); 2 g protein; 12 g carbohydrate; 2 g dietary fiber; 8 mg cholesterol; 183 mg sodium. EXCHANGE: 1½ vegetable.

Note

Six ounces of low-sodium V8 juice contains 620 mg of potassium, which helps lower blood pressure, as well as lycopene, a carotenoid that reduces risk of cancer, heart attack, and other diseases. Use only low-sodium versions of V8 and tomato juice.

Mint Julep Iced Tea

A cool, sweet, refreshing southern specialty—without the bourbon.

MAKES 4 SERVINGS   PREPARATION TIME: 1 HOUR

8 *cups water*
3 *tea bags*
2 *bunches fresh mint leaves*
¼ *cup xylitol or 6 drops stevia, to taste*
   Crushed ice

Prepare tea by bringing water just to a boil. Pour over tea bags in a large pitcher, steep for 3 to 5 minutes, remove tea bags, and chill. (Do not brew black tea for more than 5 minutes or it may become bitter.) Add xylitol and stir to dissolve.

Divide mint equally among 4 tall glasses. Place crushed ice in the glasses and pour in tea. Stir with a tall spoon to crush some of the mint leaves and serve.

PER SERVING: 33 calories; 0 g fat (0.0% calories from fat); trace protein; 13 g carbohydrate; trace dietary fiber; 0 mg cholesterol; 16 mg sodium.

SERVING IDEA: For the original mint julep, substitute bourbon and water for the tea.

Note

Mint is one of the easiest herbs to grow, either in a pot, outside or in your kitchen window, or in a corner of your garden or yard. In addition to flavoring iced tea, it's great in hot tea and makes a lovely garnish for fruit and other desserts.

Red Zinger Iced Tea

Hibiscus, rose hips, lemongrass, licorice root, and citrus
give this herbal tea its zesty flavor and rich color.

MAKES 4 SERVINGS   PREPARATION TIME: 10 MINUTES

6 cups water
3 Celestial Seasonings Red Zinger tea bags
1 tablespoon lemon juice

Bring water to a boil. Pour over tea bags and let steep for 5 minutes. Remove tea bags, add lemon juice, stir, and chill. Serve over ice.

PER SERVING: 5 calories; 0 g fat (0.0% calories from fat); trace protein; 1 g carbohydrate; trace dietary fiber; 0 mg cholesterol; 11 mg sodium.

Note
You can use any herbal or spiced tea to make flavored iced tea. Favorite flavors include peppermint, cinnamon, orange, and lemon. Sweeten with stevia, if desired.

Hot Cinnamon Cider
A nice winter party drink—keeps warm in a Crock-Pot.

MAKES 6 SERVINGS   PREPARATION TIME: 20 MINUTES

4 cups apple cider
1 cup water
5 whole allspice berries
½ teaspoon whole cloves
1 cinnamon stick

Place all ingredients in a large saucepan. Bring to a boil over medium heat. Reduce heat and simmer for 15 minutes. Strain and serve hot.

PER SERVING: 97 calories; 1 g fat (6.0% calories from fat); trace protein; 25 g carbohydrate; 3 g dietary fiber; 0 mg cholesterol; 10 mg sodium. EXCHANGES: ½ grain (starch); 1½ fruit.

Note
Scientists have discovered that cinnamon has antibacterial properties. Adding small amounts of cinnamon to apple juice contaminated with the E. coli bacteria killed 99.5 percent of the bacteria.

Perfect Green Tea

"Better to be deprived of food for three days, than tea for one."
—*ancient Chinese proverb*

MAKES 2 SERVINGS   PREPARATION TIME: 5 MINUTES

1   *teaspoon green tea*
2   *cups water plus ½ cup at room temperature*

Place loose tea in an open strainer. Do not use a tea ball, for green tea needs room to expand. Place in a small teapot or a large cup. (Make sure the teapot or cup isn't too big or the tea leaves won't sit in the water. A Japanese teapot is perfect for this. Teacups with a removable ceramic strainer are also good.)

Bring 2 cups water just to a boil, then add ½ cup room temperature water. (The ideal brewing temperature is 165 to 170 degrees F. Boiling water is too hot.)

Pour water over tea into the teapot. Steep for just 2 minutes—any longer and tea may become bitter. Do not stir.

Remove the strainer, swirl tea around, take a big whiff of the aroma, and enjoy. You may notice little flecks of tea floating around. They will settle to the bottom—and it's okay to drink them.

Do not discard the leaves. You may repeat this process 2 to 3 times with the same tea leaves, only add another minute each time to the brewing. (The second time, brew for 3 minutes, the third time, 4 minutes.)

Of course, you can also just pour not-quite-boiling water over a tea bag into a mug, steep for 2 minutes, then drink.

PER SERVING: 0 calories; 0 g fat (0.0% calories from fat); 0 g protein; 0 g carbohydrate; 0 g dietary fiber; 0 mg cholesterol; 9 mg sodium.

SERVING IDEA: Green tea is made from the same leaves as black tea, only it is not fermented. It is full of antioxidants and other protective phytonutrients that protect against heart disease, cancer, and even dental cavities! Have a cup of green tea any time you have an urge for coffee. It will perk you up, but it is lower in caffeine than other caffeinated drinks. A cup provides 30 mg of caffeine, compared to 100 mg for coffee and 50 mg for black tea.

Instant Chai

With this mix, you can have a cup of chai in minutes.

MAKES 12 SERVINGS   PREPARATION TIME: 20 MINUTES

1   cup unsweetened instant tea
1   cup nonfat dry milk powder
½   cup xylitol
1   teaspoon vanilla
1   teaspoon ground ginger
1   teaspoon ground cinnamon
½   teaspoon ground cloves
½   teaspoon ground cardamom

Combine all ingredients in a food processor or blender and process until you have a fine powder. Store in an airtight container.

To serve, stir 2 heaping tablespoons into a cup of hot water.

PER SERVING: 41 calories; trace fat (1.3% calories from fat); 2 g protein; 11 g carbohydrate; trace dietary fiber; 1 mg cholesterol; 31 mg sodium.

Note
Chai is an ancient spiced tea-milk beverage from India.

Thai Iced Coffee

Strong, bold, and different from any iced coffee you've ever tried.

MAKES 4 SERVINGS   PREPARATION TIME: 1 HOUR 15 MINUTES

6 *heaping tablespoons ground coffee*
4½ *cups water*
1 *teaspoon ground cardamom*
3 *tablespoons xylitol or 5 to 6 drops stevia, to taste*
    Ice cubes
8 *tablespoons evaporated skim milk*

Prepare coffee in a brewer, adding cardamom to ground coffee—coffee will be strong. Pour into a pitcher, stir in xylitol until it is dissolved, and cool in refrigerator, at least an hour.

Pour equal amount of cooled coffee into 4 tall glasses. Put 5 to 6 ice cubes in each glass. Pour 2 tablespoons evaporated milk into each glass.

PER SERVING: 51 calories; trace fat (0.9% calories from fat); 3 g protein; 14 g carbohydrate; 0 g dietary fiber; 1 mg cholesterol; 49 mg sodium. EXCHANGE: ½ nonfat milk.

Note

A little coffee can improve memory and focus, enhance endurance, and relieve a headache or asthma attack. Too much can not only leave you irritable and unable to sleep but contributes to osteoporosis and elevations in homocysteine levels. A cup or two (8 to 16 ounces) a day is fine; any more than that is not.

Sangria

Red wine punch from Spain.

MAKES 4 SERVINGS   PREPARATION TIME: 10 MINUTES

2 *tablespoons Cointreau*
2 *tablespoons xylitol*
½ *lemon, sliced*
½ *orange, sliced*
3 *cups dry red wine, chilled*

Mix Cointreau and xylitol in a large pitcher. Stir to dissolve xylitol. Add lemon and orange slices. Pour in wine and add ice.

PER SERVING: 174 calories; trace fat (0.6% calories from fat); 1 g protein; 14 g carbohydrate; trace dietary fiber; 0 mg cholesterol; 113 mg sodium.

Note

Alcohol used to be forbidden for diabetics. New research, however, suggests that for type 2 diabetics, moderate drinking may be associated with a reduced risk of death from heart disease. Moderation is key, and people with type 1 diabetes should avoid alcohol altogether, as should those with poorly controlled type 2 diabetes.

Hot Spiced Wine

Warms you up on a cold winter night.

MAKES 4 SERVINGS   PREPARATION TIME: 15 MINUTES

½ cup water
¼ cup xylitol
2 cinnamon sticks
5 whole cloves
2 whole allspice berries
1 orange rind, thinly sliced
1 lemon rind, thinly sliced
3 cups dry red wine

In a large saucepan, combine water, xylitol, cinnamon sticks, cloves, allspice, and orange and lemon rinds. Bring to a boil, reduce heat, and simmer for 5 minutes. Add wine and heat just to boiling. Strain and serve.

PER SERVING: 211 calories; 2 g fat (14.0% calories from fat); 1 g protein; 28 g carbohydrate; 7 g dietary fiber; 0 mg cholesterol; 138 mg sodium. EXCHANGES: 1 grain (starch); ½ fat.

Note
Red wine contains significant amounts of resveratrol, which has a number of health benefits, including antioxidant, anticoagulant, anti-inflammatory and anticancer properties.

Sandwiches and Wraps

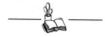

The most problematic part of a sandwich for people with diabetes is the bread. Most breads, even whole wheat breads, are made with flour. They contain a lot of carbohydrates, have a very high glycemic index, and tend to drive up blood sugar levels. Sprouted-grain breads, because they are made with whole grains rather than flour, cause a less dramatic rise in blood sugar. Sourdough bread also has a relatively low glycemic index but because it's made with white flour, we recommend it less frequently. You'll notice that many of our sandwich recipes call for only one slice of bread. Any time you can eat an open-faced sandwich, so much the better. Also, pay attention to the side dishes you eat with a sandwich. Forgo the usual high-glycemic chips and fries and have a salad, cottage cheese, or bowl of soup instead.

The sandwiches in this chapter are diverse, hearty, and healthy. Some of them, such as the Chicken Caesar Salad Wraps (page 95) and the Seafood Salad Wraps (page 96), are perfect for brown bag lunches to go. Others, such as the Chicken-Chile Quesadillas (page 108) and Grilled Vegetable–Mozzarella Panini (page 104), make an excellent main dish. And one-half of any of these sandwiches is a perfect between-meal snack. You may also use Spicy Hummus (page 58), Catalina Crab Dip (page 71), and other spreads and dips in the "Appetizers" chapter to make sandwiches.

Chicken Caesar Salad Wraps

Eat your salad without a fork—wrap it.

MAKES 4 SERVINGS   PREPARATION TIME: 10 MINUTES

4 *whole wheat tortillas*
8 *romaine leaves, plus 1⅓ cups romaine, shredded*
1½ *cups cooked chicken, coarsely chopped*
4 *tablespoons low-fat Caesar salad dressing*
8 *teaspoons grated Parmesan cheese*

Soften tortillas by heating, one at a time, in a large nonstick skillet over medium heat. Cook 30 to 60 seconds on each side, until warm and pliable.

Lay 2 romaine leaves on each tortilla, trimming if necessary to fit into tortilla. (Romaine can extend out of one end.) Spread one-fourth of shredded lettuce and chicken over center of tortilla, drizzle with 1 tablespoon dressing, and sprinkle with 2 teaspoons cheese. Wrap tightly like a burrito, folding one end under.

PER SERVING: 261 calories; 10 g fat (31.5% calories from fat); 25 g protein; 22 g carbohydrate; 1 g dietary fiber; 54 mg cholesterol; 456 mg sodium. EXCHANGES: 1½ grain (starch); 3 lean meat; 1½ fat.

SERVING IDEA: Eat these immediately or wrap them tightly in plastic wrap or foil and refrigerate.

Note
Wraps are burrito-like sandwiches with their fillings wrapped up in tortillas. They can contain most anything you can think of, from traditional sandwich fixings such as turkey slices with lettuce and tomatoes to salad ingredients as in this recipe.

Seafood Salad Wraps

A delicious shrimp and crab concoction and a snap to prepare.

MAKES 4 SERVINGS   PREPARATION TIME: 10 MINUTES

1 small (4-ounce) can tiny boiled shrimp, rinsed, drained,
  and chopped
6 ounces crabmeat (fresh or canned) or surimi (see Note, page 71),
  shredded
½ cup chopped celery
¼ cup chopped onion
⅓ cup low-fat or fat-free mayonnaise
3 tablespoons freshly chopped parsley
½ teaspoon Mrs. Dash salt-free seasoning, or to taste
⅛ teaspoon freshly ground black pepper
⅛ teaspoon garlic powder
⅛ teaspoon onion powder
4 whole wheat tortillas
8 romaine leaves

Combine shrimp, crabmeat, celery, onion, mayonnaise, parsley, and seasonings in a medium bowl and stir until well blended.

Warm tortillas by placing in a preheated skillet and heating for about 30 seconds on each side, until soft and pliable.

Place 2 romaine leaves on each tortilla and spoon one-fourth of the seafood salad over romaine. Fold an inch of tortilla up over bottom of lettuce, then tightly fold the 2 sides of tortilla across the seafood. Romaine will be poking out of the top. Wrap a napkin around the bottom of the wrap and serve.

PER SERVING: 206 calories; 7 g fat (26.9% calories from fat); 18 g protein; 24 g carbohydrate; 1 g dietary fiber; 100 mg cholesterol;

487 mg sodium. EXCHANGES: 1½ grain (starch); 2 lean meat; ½ vegetable; 1 fat.

SERVING IDEAS: Seafood Salad Wraps also make a good appetizer. Cut a wrap into 1-inch slices or serve the seafood salad with crackers or toast triangles. You may also turn it into a main dish salad by serving it on a large bed of lettuce, surrounded with tomatoes, cucumbers, green onions, and your choice of raw vegetables.

Note
Crab contains a lot of sodium, so go easy with sodium in accompanying dishes. If you are salt sensitive, double the amount of shrimp and eliminate the crab in this recipe.

Southwest Wraps

A tortilla wrapped around chicken, beans, and the works.

MAKES 4 SERVINGS   PREPARATION TIME: 10 MINUTES

1   cup cooked chicken, cut into ½-inch strips
1   cup canned black beans, rinsed and drained
4   whole wheat tortillas
8   lettuce leaves
¾   cup shredded low-sodium cheddar cheese
1   tomato, chopped
½   cup freshly chopped cilantro
¼   cup chopped onion

Heat chicken and beans in a microwave or small saucepan just until warm (not piping hot).

Warm tortillas by placing one at a time in a large nonstick skillet over medium heat. Heat for 30 to 60 seconds on each side.

Place 2 lettuce leaves on each tortilla. Spread one-fourth of chicken, beans, cheese, tomatoes, cilantro, and onion over center of each tortilla. Roll up like a burrito, tucking in bottom edge.

PER SERVING: 294 calories; 10 g fat (27.8% calories from fat); 24 g protein; 33 g carbohydrate; 5 g dietary fiber; 51 mg cholesterol; 415 mg sodium. EXCHANGES: 2 grain (starch); 2½ lean meat; ½ vegetable; 1 fat.

SERVING IDEA: Serve this with Mary's Fresh Salsa (page 283) or Quick and Easy Salsa (page 284). If you want to splurge, add Guacamole (page 55).

Crunchy Tuna Sandwiches

Celery and almonds give this sandwich filling a crunch.

MAKES 4 SERVINGS   PREPARATION TIME: 10 MINUTES

1 small can tuna in water (6 ounces, preferably albacore), drained
¼ cup low-fat or fat-free mayonnaise
⅛ teaspoon seasoned salt or salt substitute
⅛ teaspoon freshly ground black pepper
½ cup chopped celery
½ cup chopped apple
2 tablespoons chopped onion
¼ cup chopped almonds
4 slices sprouted-grain bread
4 large tomato slices

Combine first seven ingredients in a medium bowl. Mix well. Stir in almonds just before serving. Serve open-faced on 4 pieces of sprouted-grain bread, topping each with slice of tomato.

PER SERVING: 238 calories; 10 g fat (35.9% calories from fat); 17 g protein; 22 g carbohydrate; 5 g dietary fiber; 18 mg cholesterol; 348 mg sodium. EXCHANGES: 1 grain (starch); 2 lean meat; ½ vegetable; 1½ fat.

Note
Limit tuna to 1 can a week. Canned tuna may contain unsafe levels of mercury, which is a neurological toxin.

Healthy Clubs

*The only thing missing from this classic club sandwich
is excess saturated fat and calories.*

MAKES 4 SERVINGS   PREPARATION TIME: 20 MINUTES

6 slices turkey bacon or vegetarian bacon (see Note)
8 slices sprouted-grain bread
4 tablespoons fat-free or low-fat mayonnaise
6 ounces cooked turkey breast meat or chicken breast meat
1 large tomato, sliced
4 small lettuce leaves

Heat a large nonstick skillet over medium heat. Place turkey bacon in
a single layer in the skillet and cook, turning as needed, until crisp,
about 5 minutes. Drain on paper towels. (Or cook in microwave.)

Toast bread slices.

Spread mayonnaise on one side of each slice of bread. Evenly
divide and arrange turkey breast on 4 slices. Place 1½ pieces of
turkey bacon on each, then tomato slices and lettuce leaf, and top
with piece of bread.

PER SERVING: 311 calories; 8 g fat (24.2% calories from fat); 24 g
protein; 35 g carbohydrate; 6 g dietary fiber; 50 mg cholesterol;
647 mg sodium. EXCHANGES: 2 grain (starch); 3 lean meat; ½ vegetable; ½ fat.

Note

Vegetarian bacon is a reasonable substitute and contains less
sodium. Good brands are Morningstar Farms Breakfast Strips and
Worthington Stripples.

Smoked Salmon Sandwiches

Buy smoked salmon fresh or vacuum-sealed.

MAKES 4 SERVINGS   PREPARATION TIME: 10 MINUTES

8 *ounces smoked salmon*
4 *slices pumpernickel bread*
4 *very thin slices red onion*
4 *teaspoons capers (optional)*

Place thin slices of smoked salmon on each slice of bread. Top with onion slices and 1 teaspoon capers per sandwich. Serve open-faced.

PER SERVING: 207 calories; 4 g fat (15.9% calories from fat); 15 g protein; 29 g carbohydrate; 5 g dietary fiber; 13 mg cholesterol; 690 mg sodium. EXCHANGES: 1 grain (starch); 1½ lean meat; 2½ vegetable.

SERVING IDEA: Serve these for lunch, along with 21st-Century Waldorf Salad (page 123) or another salad.

Note
Smoked salmon is high in sodium. Cut serving size down to 1 ounce, if desired.

Grilled Turkey Sandwiches

A George Foreman grill is great for grilling sandwiches.

MAKES 4 SERVINGS   PREPARATION TIME: 20 MINUTES

8 *slices pumpernickel bread*
   Olive oil spray
2 *ounces low-sodium Swiss cheese*
4 *ounces low-sodium turkey slices*
4 *teaspoons Mac's Special Sauce (page 281) or mustard*
1 *small tomato, sliced*
4 *red onion slices*
4 *lettuce leaves*

Heat a nonstick griddle, large skillet, or George Foreman grill over medium heat. Spray one side of bread with olive oil spray and place on griddle, skillet, or grill sprayed side down. Place cheese and turkey on bread and top with another slice of bread. Spray top piece of bread with olive oil. Cook until bread is browned; turn, and continue cooking until other side is browned and cheese has melted. This will only take 3 to 5 minutes per side—or 3 to 5 minutes total if you're using a George Foreman grill.

Open and spread each with 1 teaspoon Mac's Special Sauce. Add tomato and red onion slices and lettuce and close.

PER SERVING (includes Mac's Special Sauce): 268 calories; 8 g fat (27% calories from fat); 16 g protein; 34 g carbohydrate; 5 g dietary fiber; 30 mg cholesterol; 457 mg sodium. EXCHANGES: 2 grain (starch); 1½ lean meat; ½ vegetable; 1 fat.

Note

Prepared lunch meats are often loaded with sodium nitrites and other additives. Look for low-fat, low-sodium brands of turkey, turkey pastrami, and other favorites.

Gourmet PB&Js

Spruce up peanut butter and jelly on the griddle.

MAKES 4 SERVINGS   PREPARATION TIME: 15 MINUTES

4 tablespoons peanut butter *(natural, without hydrogenated oils)*
8 teaspoons fruit-juice sweetened jam *(not jelly)*
8 slices sprouted-grain bread
   Olive oil spray

Spread 1 tablespoon of peanut butter and 2 teaspoons of jam over 1 slice of bread. Top with another slice. Repeat with remaining bread.

Heat a nonstick griddle or large skillet over medium heat. Spray both sides of sandwiches with olive oil spray and cook 2 to 4 minutes on each side, until golden brown. (Or use a George Foreman grill and cook until lightly browned.)

PER SERVING: 288 calories; 9 g fat (28% calories from fat); 12 g protein; 42 g carbohydrate; 7 g dietary fiber; 0 mg cholesterol; 231 mg sodium. EXCHANGES: 2 grain (starch); 1½ lean meat; 1½ fat; 1 other carbohydrate.

SERVING IDEA: To lower carbohydrate count, use one piece of bread per serving.

Note

Harvard researchers found that women who ate a small serving of peanut butter and/or nuts at least five times a week had a 27 percent lower risk of developing diabetes than those who rarely ate nuts. Yes, peanut butter is high in fat, but it's unsaturated fat, which helps improve blood sugar and insulin control.

Grilled Vegetable–Mozzarella Panini

Paninis are thin, grilled Italian sandwiches, and this one's a dandy.

MAKES 4 SERVINGS   PREPARATION TIME: 35 MINUTES

Olive oil spray
1½ cups sliced mushrooms
 1 medium zucchini, sliced lengthwise into ¼-inch strips
 1 medium red onion, thinly sliced
 1 tablespoon extra-virgin olive oil
 2 cloves garlic, peeled and minced
 ½ teaspoon dried tarragon
 ¼ teaspoon seasoned salt or salt substitute
 ¼ teaspoon freshly ground black pepper
 8 slices sourdough bread, thinly sliced
 4 ounces part skim milk mozzarella cheese, thinly sliced

Preheat the oven to 475 degrees F. Spray a 9-by-13-inch baking dish with olive oil spray.

Place mushrooms, zucchini, and red onion slices in the baking dish. Mix olive oil, garlic, tarragon, salt, and pepper in a small bowl, then brush over vegetables. Bake for 10 to 15 minutes, until soft. (You may also grill or broil vegetables, about 5 minutes on each side.)

Heat a nonstick griddle, large skillet, or George Foreman grill over medium heat.

Spray 1 side of each slice of bread with olive oil spray. Spread one-fourth of the cheese and vegetables over unsprayed side of a slice of bread. Place another slice, sprayed side up, on top. Repeat with remaining slices.

Heat sandwiches on the griddle, pressing down with a spatula, until golden brown, about 3 to 5 minutes. Turn and cook other side until brown and cheese melts. (A George Foreman grill works particularly well for panini and requires no turnings.)

PER SERVING: 285 calories; 10 g fat (31.4% calories from fat); 14 g protein; 36 g carbohydrate; 4 g dietary fiber; 15 mg cholesterol; 545 mg sodium. EXCHANGES: 2 grain (starch); 1 lean meat; 1½ vegetable; 1 fat.

SERVING IDEA: Serve with Dijon mustard or to really jazz these sandwiches up, spread on a little Black Olive Tapenade (page 66) or Pesto (page 296).

Note
Because of its acidity, sourdough bread causes a less dramatic rise in blood sugar than most breads. If you can find whole wheat sourdough bread, go for it. You may also use sprouted-grain bread.

Falafel Sandwiches with Garlic Sauce

*This Middle Eastern delicacy is baked, not fried,
and topped with a tangy yogurt-garlic sauce.*

MAKES 8 SERVINGS   PREPARATION TIME: 20 MINUTES

Olive oil spray
1 (15-ounce) can garbanzo beans, rinsed and drained
1 egg white or ⅛ cup Egg Beaters or other egg white product
1 tablespoon tahini (see Note, page 58)
¼ cup minced onion
4 tablespoons freshly chopped parsley
2 cloves garlic, peeled and minced
1 teaspoon ground cumin
½ teaspoon ground coriander
¼ teaspoon freshly ground black pepper
4 rounds whole wheat pita bread
2 tomatoes, chopped
1 cucumber, chopped
2 cups shredded lettuce
1 cup Garlic Sauce (page 287)

Preheat the oven to 400 degrees F. Spray a cookie sheet with olive oil spray.

Process beans in a food processor or blender until smooth, or mash with a fork. Transfer to a medium bowl.

Add egg white, tahini, onion, parsley, garlic, cumin, coriander, and pepper. Stir until well blended.

Scoop rounded tablespoons of mixture onto the prepared cookie sheet. Flatten and shape with your hands into 8 flat patties.

Bake for 6 minutes. Remove from the oven, turn, and bake an additional 5 to 8 minutes, until heated through and lightly browned.

Cut pita bread rounds in half. Place 1 falafel in each half and stuff with tomatoes, cucumbers, and lettuce. Serve with Garlic Sauce.

PER SERVING (includes Garlic Sauce): 226 calories; 4 g fat (13.8% calories from fat); 11 g protein; 40 g carbohydrate; 8 g dietary fiber; 1 mg cholesterol; 280 mg sodium. EXCHANGES: 2 grain (starch); ½ lean meat; ½ vegetable; ½ fat.

SERVING IDEA: You can also serve falafel as an appetizer or snack. Shape them into smaller patties and serve with Garlic Sauce. (They are rather dry, and the Garlic Sauce perks them up.)

Chicken-Chile Quesadillas
A sandwich from south of the border.

MAKES 4 SERVINGS   PREPARATION TIME: 10 MINUTES

  4 ounces cooked chicken
  4 large whole wheat tortillas
  4 ounces Monterey Jack cheese, grated
  ½ small (4-ounce) can chopped green chiles, well drained

Heat cooked chicken in a microwave for about 1 minute (or wrap in foil and heat in a preheated 350 degree F oven for 10 minutes), until warm.

Heat a large nonstick skillet over medium heat. Place 1 tortilla in the skillet and heat until warm. Turn tortilla over so cooked side is up and spread one-quarter of the cheese, chicken, and chiles over one half the tortilla. Fold the empty half of the tortilla over the filling. Cook over medium heat until tortilla turns golden brown and cheese begins to melt. Flip and cook other side until golden brown. Repeat with other tortillas and remaining cheese, chicken, and chiles. Cut in half and serve.

PER SERVING: 231 calories; 10 g fat (36.9% calories from fat); 19 g protein; 21 g carbohydrate; trace dietary fiber; 49 mg cholesterol; 346 mg sodium. EXCHANGES: 1½ grain (starch); 2 lean meat; 1 fat,

SERVING IDEAS: Serve these with Quick and Easy Salsa (page 284) or Mary's Fresh Salsa (page 283). Makes a nice light meal along with a salad, or an appetizer, cut into small wedges.

Healthy "Hamburgers"
Who says hamburgers can't be healthy?

MAKES 4 SERVINGS   PREPARATION TIME: 30 MINUTES

4 soy burger patties (see Note)
2 whole hamburger buns, preferably sprouted-grain
4 slices red onion
4 lettuce leaves
1 medium tomato, sliced
4 tablespoons Mac's Special Sauce (page 281)

Cook soy burgers per package instructions. You can also cook them on the grill. They just need to be heated through. Be careful not to overcook them or they'll get hard.

Place each burger on half a bun. Top with red onion slice, lettuce leaf, tomato slices, and Mac's Special Sauce. Eat with a knife and fork.

PER SERVING (includes Mac's Special Sauce): 232 calories; 4 g fat (58% calories from fat); 17 g protein; 35 g carbohydrate; 8 g dietary fiber; 0 mg cholesterol; 405 mg sodium. EXCHANGES: 1 grain (starch); 2 lean meat; 2½ vegetable; ½ fat.

SERVING IDEA: To cut back on carbs, we're suggesting that you eat this burger open-faced (with half of a bun)—or with no bun at all.

Note
Good brands of soy-based vegetarian hamburger patties include Boca burgers, which come in assorted flavors such as roasted garlic, Morningstar Farms Grillers, Flame Grilled Hamburger Style Gardenburgers, and Amy's All America. Nutritional analysis will vary depending on brand.

Patty Melts

A vegetarian version of an all-American favorite.

MAKES 4 SERVINGS   PREPARATION TIME: 25 MINUTES

1   teaspoon extra-virgin olive oil
1   medium onion, sliced
2   tablespoons water
4   soy burger patties (see Note, page 109)
4   slices rye bread
    Olive oil spray
2   ounces low-sodium Swiss cheese, thinly sliced

Heat olive oil over medium heat in a large nonstick skillet. Add onion slices and cook, stirring occasionally, for 2 minutes. Turn heat down, add 2 tablespoons water, cover, and cook 5 minutes, until soft. Turn up heat and cook until golden brown, about 3 minutes. Remove from skillet and keep warm.

Meanwhile, prepare soy burgers per package instructions.

Return the skillet to the stove and heat over medium heat. Spray both sides of bread slices with olive oil spray. Brown bread in the skillet, turning after about 2 minutes, or until lightly toasted.

Preheat the broiler.

Place 1 burger on each slice of bread. Divide grilled onions evenly on burgers. Top with cheese. Place on a cookie sheet and cook under the broiler until cheese melts, 1 to 2 minutes.

PER SERVING: 257 calories; 8 g fat (27.8% calories from fat); 20 g protein; 27 g carbohydrate; 6 g dietary fiber; 13 mg cholesterol; 484 mg sodium. EXCHANGES: 1½ grain (starch); 2½ lean meat; ½ vegetable; 1½ fat.

Sloppy Josés

A Mexican twist on a favorite sandwich.

MAKES 4 SERVINGS   PREPARATION TIME: 30 MINUTES

1 *pound lean ground turkey*
½ *cup chopped onion*
½ *cup chopped green bell pepper*
12 *ounces chili sauce or tomato sauce*
1½ *tablespoon Worcestershire sauce*
2 *teaspoons chili powder or to taste*
¼ *teaspoon red pepper flakes, or to taste*
2 *hamburger buns, preferably sprouted-grain*

Heat a large nonstick skillet over medium heat. Add ground turkey, onion, and green pepper and cook, stirring often with a wooden spoon to break up turkey meat. Cook until turkey is done (no longer pink), about 10 minutes.

Stir in chili sauce, Worcestershire sauce, chili powder, and red pepper flakes. Bring to a boil, reduce heat, and simmer for 5 to 10 minutes, stirring occasionally, until most of the liquid has evaporated.

Pile turkey on top of hamburger bun halves and serve open-faced.

PER SERVING: 262 calories; 10 g fat (31.8% calories from fat); 26 g protein; 20 g carbohydrate; 3 g dietary fiber; 73 mg cholesterol; 291 mg sodium. EXCHANGES: 1 grain (starch); 3½ lean meat; ½ vegetable; ½ fat; ½ other carbohydrates.

SERVING IDEA: Sloppy Josés are so messy they're better eaten with a fork.

Note
For traditional Sloppy Joes, omit the chili powder.

Smart Hot Dogs

*You'll be surprised at how good veggie hot dogs taste,
especially when smothered in chili or sauerkraut.*

MAKES 4 SERVINGS   PREPARATION TIME: 20 MINUTES

1   cup Chipotle Chili (page 140) or low-sodium, low-fat canned chili
4   soy dogs (see Notes)
4   hot dog buns, preferably sprouted-grain
4   teaspoons mustard
¼   cup chopped onion

Heat chili in a small saucepan over medium heat, about 5 minutes.

Heat hot dogs per package instructions. You can grill soy dogs, but take care not to overcook them. And watch out—they cook fast, so just heat them through.

Place 1 hot dog in each bun, spread mustard over hot dog, and top with ¼ cup chili and sprinkling of chopped onion.

PER SERVING (includes chili): 248 calories; 3 g fat (11.2% calories from fat); 18 g protein; 34 g carbohydrate; 5 g dietary fiber; 0 mg cholesterol; 758 mg sodium. EXCHANGES: 2 grain (starch); 2 lean meat; ½ vegetable; ½ fat.

SERVING IDEAS: The sodium content will be dramatically reduced if you use Chipotle Chili or low-sodium canned chili. Nevertheless, the veggie dogs have 400 mg sodium each, so if you are salt sensitive, this recipe might not be for you. Also good with sauerkraut (again, salt sensitives beware).

Notes

A 2002 Harvard study found that men who ate hot dogs and other processed meats such as bacon and bologna more than five times a week had twice the risk of developing type 2 diabetes than those who ate these foods less frequently.

Good brands of soy dogs are Yves Veggie Cuisines, Worthington Leanies, and Lightlife Meatless Smart Dogs. Nutritional analysis will vary somewhat, depending on brand and size.

Salads

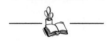

Salads have moved far beyond bland mixtures of iceberg lettuce, grated carrots, pale tomatoes, and bottled salad dressing. We guarantee you'll find the recipes in this chapter to be anything but bland. Among the many attributes of salads is that they are extremely nutritious. Tomatoes, onions, spinach, lettuces, and other vegetables and leafy greens contain a cornucopia of health-enhancing antioxidants, fiber, minerals, and phytonutrients. They are also low in calories and have an extremely low glycemic index, making them ideal foods for people with diabetes. (What you add to your salads may be another story—but not in the case of these recipes. You can enjoy them without worrying about your blood sugar or your waistline.)

Another attribute of salads is ease of preparation. Many of our salads can be made in minutes. The rest can be prepared ahead of time and refrigerated, making them convenient for those days when you just don't have time to cook. Fully half of the recipes in this chapter, such as Shrimp Louie (page 121) and Chicken and Wild Rice Salad (page 117), are hearty and balanced enough to serve as entrées. In addition to the salad recipes here, keep in mind that many of the grilled, broiled, or sautéed shrimp, fish, and poultry dishes in this cookbook can be turned into entrée salads—just serve on a bed of greens with your favorite salad dressing.

A note of interest to people with diabetes: the acids in vinegar, lemon, and lime slow the emptying of food from the stomach and thus retard the release of blood sugar. Eating as little as three or four teaspoons of an acidic food lowers the glycemic index of the meal and helps keep blood sugar levels in check. So green salads with oil and vinegar/lemon/lime dressing actually help with blood sugar control. (The same blood sugar–lowering effect is true for other acidic foods such as yogurt and buttermilk.)

This may go without saying, but always wash fresh produce (organic included) well just before using. Simply rinsing under cold running water and rubbing with your hands removes dirt, pesticides, and bacteria. You may use a brush to scrub carrots, potatoes, and other tough-skinned produce, as well as the rinds of lemon, limes, and melons before cutting.

BLT Salad

If you like bacon, lettuce, and tomato sandwiches,
you'll love this salad.

MAKES 4 LARGE SERVINGS (8 CUPS)   PREPARATION TIME: 15 MINUTES

6 slices turkey bacon or soy bacon
6 cups coarsely chopped romaine lettuce
3 medium tomatoes, coarsely chopped
½ cup Farm Dressing and Dip (page 276) or reduced-fat ranch
   dressing
   Dash freshly ground black pepper
   Dash salt

Cook bacon per package instructions. Cool and chop.

Combine bacon, romaine, and tomatoes in a large bowl. Toss with dressing, add salt and pepper, and serve.

PER SERVING (includes dressing): 127 calories; 8 g fat (50.6% calories from fat); 8 g protein; 12 g carbohydrate; 3 g dietary fiber; 28 mg cholesterol; 403 mg sodium. EXCHANGES: ½ lean meat; 1½ vegetable; 1 fat.

Chicken and Wild Rice Salad
A hearty main dish salad.

MAKES 4 SERVINGS (5 CUPS)   PREPARATION TIME: 1 HOUR 30 MINUTES

½ *cup wild rice*
1¼ *cups low-sodium chicken broth (optional) or water*
2 *tablespoons hazelnut oil or extra-virgin olive oil*
1 *tablespoon apple cider vinegar*
1 *teaspoon xylitol or brown rice syrup*
½ *teaspoon Low-Sodium Seasoned Salt (page 297) or salt substitute*
½ *teaspoon freshly ground black pepper*
1½ *cups cooked chicken, chopped into bite-sized pieces (see Notes)*
¼ *cup chopped green bell peppers*
¼ *cup thinly sliced or chopped green onions*
¼ *cup grated carrot*
½ *cup dried cranberries or dried apricots*
¼ *cup chopped pecans*
8 *lettuce leaves*

At least an hour and a half before serving, cook wild rice per package directions. (Bring chicken broth to a boil in a medium saucepan. Add rice, return to a boil, then turn down heat, cover, and simmer for 45 to 50 minutes, or until kernels begin to puff open. Turn heat off and let sit, covered, for 10 minutes. Uncover, drain off excess liquid, and fluff with a fork.) Place in a serving bowl and cool in refrigerator for at least 15 minutes.

Meanwhile, mix hazelnut oil, vinegar, xylitol, salt, and pepper in a small bowl.

(continued)

Chicken and Wild Rice Salad *(continued)*

Add chicken to wild rice, along with green peppers, green onions, carrot, cranberries, and pecans. Pour oil and vinegar mixture over wild rice mixture and mix well. Serve at room temperature or chilled.

To serve, place 2 lettuce leaves on each of four serving plates. Spoon wild rice mixture onto lettuce.

PER SERVING: 300 calories; 14 g fat (41% calories from fat); 24 g protein; 21 g carbohydrate; 3 g dietary fiber; 45 mg cholesterol; 413 mg sodium. EXCHANGES: 1 grain (starch); 2½ lean meat; ½ vegetable; 2½ fat.

Notes

There are several ways to cook chicken breast(s). Defrost (use a microwave if you're in a hurry), then boil for about 10 minutes. Cutting chicken into smaller pieces reduces cooking time. You can also sauté chicken in a little olive oil for 10 to 12 minutes, turning once, or cook in a George Foreman grill for 6 to 7 minutes (it will be drier). To test for doneness, cut into the thickest area—there should be no pinkness and juices should be clear.

If your recipe calls for chilled chicken, you can hasten the cooling process by placing cooked chicken in the freezer for 20 to 30 minutes. Cooked chicken will keep in the refrigerator for about a week, so cook an extra breast or two to use in other recipes or to eat as a snack.

Chicken-Grape Salad

An oldie but goodie.

MAKES 4 SERVINGS (4 CUPS) PREPARATION TIME: 1 HOUR 10 MINUTES

2 cups cooked chicken *(see Notes, page 118)*
2 stalks celery, chopped
1 cup halved seedless grapes
½ cup low-fat or fat-free mayonnaise
½ teaspoon dried thyme
¼ teaspoon salt or salt substitute
¼ teaspoon freshly ground black pepper
8 romaine leaves

Cut cooked chicken into bite-sized pieces.

Mix chicken, celery, and grapes together in a large bowl.

Combine mayonnaise, thyme, salt, and pepper in a small bowl and mix well. Stir into chicken mixture until moist and creamy.

Refrigerate covered for at least 1 hour before serving.

Serve on romaine leaves.

PER SERVING: 232 calories; 11 g fat (44.5% calories from fat); 22 g protein; 10 g carbohydrate; 1 g dietary fiber; 70 mg cholesterol; 351 mg sodium. EXCHANGES: 3 lean meat; ½ fruit; 1½ fat.

SERVING IDEAS: Serve this as a main dish, along with a bowl of vegetable soup. It also makes a good sandwich or wrap filling. Simply chop chicken and grapes coarsely, then proceed with recipe.

Luscious Layered Salad

A make-ahead salad that everyone loves.

MAKES 6 SERVINGS (9 CUPS)   PREPARATION TIME: 1 HOUR 15 MINUTES

6 cups coarsely chopped romaine lettuce
1 (10-ounce) package frozen peas, defrosted
⅓ cup low-fat mayonnaise
½ teaspoon Low-Sodium Seasoned Salt (page 297) or salt substitute
2 stalks celery, thinly sliced
4 green onions (with green tops), thinly sliced
1 large tomato, chopped
3 slices turkey bacon, cooked and crumbled, or 6 tablespoons soy
   bacon bits
¾ cup grated sharp Cheddar cheese

Place romaine in a medium salad bowl. Spread peas evenly over romaine. Spread mayonnaise evenly over peas, and sprinkle salt over mayonnaise.

Layer remaining ingredients evenly over peas and mayonnaise in this order: celery, onions, tomato, turkey bacon, and cheese.

Cover and refrigerate at least 1 hour before serving.

PER SERVING: 164 calories; 10 g fat (53% calories from fat); 8 g protein; 11 g carbohydrate; 4 g dietary fiber; 26 mg cholesterol; 429 mg sodium. EXCHANGES: ½ grain (starch); ½ lean meat; ½ vegetable; 1½ fruit; 1 fat.

SERVING IDEA: Show off this layered creation by serving it in a clear salad bowl. To serve, scoop straight down in bowl to get all layers.

Shrimp Louie

*Legend is that this recipe was created for Enrico Caruso
at Seattle's Olympic Hotel.*

MAKES 4 SERVINGS (11 CUPS)   PREPARATION TIME: 20 MINUTES

12 ounces (36 to 45) cooked small shrimp (canned, fresh, or frozen)
 8 cups romaine lettuce, torn into bite-sized pieces
 2 large tomatoes, cut into ½-inch wedges
 ½ cup chopped red onion
 4 hard-boiled egg whites, sliced into thin wedges
 ½ avocado, cut into 1-inch slices
 ½ cup ripe olives, drained
 ¾ cup Louie Salad Dressing (page 277)

Rinse shrimp in cold water and drain.

Place romaine on individual serving plates. Divide shrimp and pile in the middle of romaine. Arrange one-fourth of the tomato wedges, red onion, egg white wedges, avocado, and olives in a circular pattern around shrimp on each plate. Pour dressing evenly over the top.

PER SERVING (includes Louie Dressing): 309 calories; 17 g fat (49.5% calories from fat); 24 g protein; 14 g carbohydrate; 4 g dietary fiber; 180 mg cholesterol; 612 mg sodium. EXCHANGES: 3 lean meat; 1½ vegetable; 3 fat.

SERVING IDEA: Serve this as a main dish with a cup of Manhattan Clam Chowder (page 153) on the side.

Note
Actually, the original Louie was a Crab Louie. Replace the shrimp with ¾ pound cooked, flaked crabmeat (or surimi) if you want to try the original.

Zesty Cottage Cheese
A different way to serve cottage cheese.

MAKES 4 SERVINGS (2 CUPS)   PREPARATION TIME: 2 HOURS 10 MINUTES

1½ cups low-fat cottage cheese
2 tablespoons chopped red onion
¼ cup chopped radishes
¼ cup canned chopped green chiles, drained

Combine all ingredients in a medium bowl. Mix well, cover, and refrigerate for at least 2 hours.

PER SERVING: 69 calories; 1 g fat (12.4% calories from fat); 11 g protein; 4 g carbohydrate; trace dietary fiber; 4 mg cholesterol; 347 mg sodium. EXCHANGES: 1½ lean meat; ½ vegetable.

SERVING IDEAS: Try it with other additions, such as chopped green onions or chives, or diced fruit (peaches and apricots are particularly good).

Note
Low-fat or nonfat cottage cheese is an extremely versatile source of protein. In addition to being a salad ingredient, it is a good between-meal snack that won't wreak havoc with your blood sugar levels. It can also be blended and turned into a dip or sandwich spread, and it cuts back on fat when used in place of cheese in quiches and casseroles.

21st-Century Waldorf Salad
A healthy update on an old favorite.

MAKES 4 SERVINGS (4 CUPS)   PREPARATION TIME: 15 MINUTES

⅓ cup low-fat mayonnaise
1 teaspoon lemon juice
1 Granny Smith apple
1 red apple (preferably Fuji)
½ cup chopped celery
½ cup chopped radishes
¼ cup chopped red onion
¼ cup dried cranberries
¼ cup chopped pecans

Mix mayonnaise and lemon juice.

Core apples (do not peel) and chop into ½-inch pieces.

Combine apples, celery, radishes, red onion, and cranberries in a large bowl and add mayonnaise, stirring well to coat. Cover and refrigerate.

Just before serving, stir in pecans.

PER SERVING: 144 calories; 10 g fat (60.7% calories from fat); 1 g protein; 14 g carbohydrate; 3 g dietary fiber; 7 mg cholesterol; 112 mg sodium. EXCHANGES: ½ vegetable; ½ fruit; 2 fat.

SERVING IDEA: Serve this on a bed of lettuce.

Note
Dried cranberries and radishes give this Waldorf salad a unique flavor.

Cabbage and Carrot Slaw

Fat-free, crunchy, and loaded with nutrients.

MAKES 4 SERVINGS (5 CUPS)   PREPARATION TIME: 20 MINUTES

4 cups (about ½ medium head) chopped cabbage
1 cup grated carrots
¼ cup chopped onion
½ cup fat-free or low-fat mayonnaise
2 tablespoons skim milk
2 tablespoons chopped parsley
2 teaspoons Mrs. Dash salt-free seasoning
¼ teaspoon Low-Sodium Seasoned Salt (page 297)
¼ teaspoon lemon pepper

Combine cabbage, carrots, and onion in a large bowl.

Mix mayonnaise, milk, parsley, and seasonings together in a small bowl and stir well.

Pour dressing over cabbage mixture and stir until blended.

PER SERVING: 68 calories; trace fat (4.3% calories from fat); 2 g protein; 16 g carbohydrate; 3 g dietary fiber; trace cholesterol; 519 mg sodium. EXCHANGE: 1½ vegetable.

Note
Raw cabbage has long been used to treat indigestion and ulcers. Drinking 1 quart of cabbage juice (purchased, extracted in a juicer, or pulverized in a blender or food processor with water) a day for 10 days has been shown in clinical studies to completely heal peptic ulcers. The high glutamine content in cabbage strengthens the lining of the stomach and intestinal tract.

Blue Cheese Lovers' Salad

The name says it all.

MAKES 4 SERVINGS (7 CUPS)   PREPARATION TIME: 10 MINUTES

6 cups lettuce (*preferably mixed baby greens*)
1 pear or apple, cored and very thinly sliced
¼ cup thinly sliced red onion
4 tablespoons crumbled blue cheese
4 tablespoons Basic Vinaigrette (*page 274*)

Wash lettuce, tear into bite-sized pieces, and divide equally on four small serving plates.

Arrange pear and onion slices on top of lettuce. Sprinkle 1 tablespoon blue cheese over each salad.

Top each salad with 1 tablespoon Basic Vinaigrette.

PER SERVING (includes Basic Vinaigrette): 129 calories; 9 g fat (61.9% calories from fat); 3 g protein; 10 g carbohydrate; 3 g dietary fiber; 5 mg cholesterol; 193 mg sodium. EXCHANGES: ½ vegetable; ½ fruit; 2 fat.

Note
Blue cheese is so named for its ribbons of blue mold. Roquefort cheese (France), Stilton (England), Gorgonzola (Italy), Danablu (Denmark), and Maytag Blue (U.S.) are a few varieties.

Island Breeze Salad

The fragrance of lime hints of the islands.

2 *tablespoons lime juice*
2 *tablespoons xylitol*
2 *teaspoons macadamia oil or almond oil*
¼ *teaspoon freshly ground black pepper*
   Pinch ground ginger
6 *cups lettuce: leaf, romaine, or mixed greens*
¼ *cup thinly sliced onion (preferably sweet Maui)*
2 *kiwifruit, peeled and thinly sliced*
¼ *cup macadamia nuts or blanched almonds*

Mix lime juice, xylitol, macadamia or almond oil, pepper, and ginger in a small bowl. Set aside.

In a large bowl, toss lettuce with onion slices and kiwifruit. Pour in lime juice mixture and toss to coat evenly. Add nuts and toss again.

PER SERVING: 138 calories; 9 g fat (50.4% calories from fat); 2 g protein; 17 g carbohydrate; 4 g dietary fiber; 0 mg cholesterol; 10 mg sodium. EXCHANGES: ½ vegetable; ½ fruit; 1½ fat.

Note

Citrus fruit is a great source of vitamin C. Scurvy, caused by vitamin C deficiencies, killed more British seamen than any other enemy until the early 1800s, when vitamin C–rich lime juice was added to their daily rations (which included rum).

Curried Quinoa Salad

The combination of quinoa and curry provides unbeatable health benefits.

MAKES 4 SERVINGS (4 CUPS)   PREPARATION TIME: 30 MINUTES

- 1 cup low-sodium chicken broth
- 1 tablespoon curry powder
- ½ cup quinoa
- 2 teaspoons extra-virgin olive oil
- 1 tablespoon lemon juice
- ¼ teaspoon Low-Sodium Seasoned Salt (page 297) or salt substitute
- ¼ teaspoon freshly ground black pepper
- ½ cup finely chopped carrot
- ½ cup finely chopped celery
- ½ cup finely chopped zucchini
- ¼ cup finely chopped onion
- 1 small tomato, finely chopped
- 2 tablespoons finely chopped dried apricots
- ¼ cup chopped peanuts

Bring chicken broth and curry powder to a boil in a medium saucepan.

Rinse quinoa well and drain. Stir into boiling broth, reduce heat and simmer for 15 to 20 minutes.

Mix olive oil, lemon juice, salt, and pepper in a small bowl.

Transfer quinoa to a large bowl and fluff up with a fork. Add vegetables and apricots, and stir in oil-lemon mixture. Stir with a fork until all ingredients are well blended. Cover and refrigerate until ready to serve.

(continued)

Curried Quinoa Salad *(continued)*

Sprinkle peanuts over salad just before serving.

PER SERVING: 202 calories; 8 g fat (35.4% calories from fat); 9 g protein; 25 g carbohydrate; 4 g dietary fiber; 0 mg cholesterol; 245 mg sodium. EXCHANGES: 1 grain (starch); ½ lean meat; 1 vegetable; 1½ fat.

SERVING IDEAS: This is good cold or at room temperature. Turn it into a main dish salad by stirring in 1 cup diced cooked chicken breast. Or top individual servings with a fillet of grilled fish.

Note

Eat curry often. One of the herbs in curry powder, turmeric, contains an ingredient called curcumin. It is being studied for its ability to reduce inflammation and amyloid deposits in the brain, key features of Alzheimer's disease.

Salade à la Grecque

Feta and olives liven up this salad.

MAKES 4 SERVINGS (10 CUPS)   PREPARATION TIME: 15 MINUTES

2 tablespoons extra-virgin olive oil
2 tablespoons balsamic vinegar
1 clove garlic, peeled and minced
¼ teaspoon Low-Sodium Seasoned Salt (page 297) or salt substitute
¼ teaspoon freshly ground black pepper
8 cups romaine lettuce, torn into bite-sized pieces
1 small tomato, cut into thin wedges
½ small cucumber, sliced
⅓ cup very thinly sliced onion (preferably sweet Maui)
⅓ cup black pitted olives (preferably kalamata)
¼ cup crumbled feta cheese

Prepare salad dressing by mixing olive oil, vinegar, garlic, salt, and pepper.

Combine all salad ingredients, including olives and cheese, in a large bowl. Toss with dressing and serve.

PER SERVING: 144 calories; 11 g fat (60.2% calories from fat); 5 g protein; 10 g carbohydrate; 5 g dietary fiber; 8 mg cholesterol; 308 mg sodium. EXCHANGES: 1½ vegetable; 2 fat.

SERVING IDEA: Turn this into a main dish by topping with 1 pound sautéed or grilled shrimp (4 ounces per serving).

Note

It's worth your while to seek out kalamata olives. These firm black olives from the Kalamata area of Greece are aged for at least 3 months, giving them a unique, intense flavor.

Orange County Special

Chockfull of vitamin C and beta-carotene.

MAKES 4 SERVINGS (8 CUPS)   PREPARATION TIME: 15 MINUTES

1½ tablespoons extra-virgin olive oil
1½ tablespoons red wine vinegar or lemon juice
  1 teaspoon finely chopped parsley
  ¼ teaspoon salt or salt substitute
  ¼ teaspoon freshly ground black pepper
  6 cups lettuce (preferably mixed baby greens) or romaine
  2 oranges
  ½ small red onion, peeled and very thinly sliced
  2 teaspoons freshly chopped parsley, for garnish

Make salad dressing by mixing olive oil, vinegar, parsley, salt, and pepper in a small bowl.

Wash lettuce and tear into bite-sized pieces. Divide evenly among four small serving plates or salad bowls.

Peel oranges, carefully cut away white pith, and cut into ¼-inch slices. Arrange slices from half an orange on each plate of lettuce.

Divide onion slices and arrange on orange slices.

Spoon salad dressing over salads. Garnish with parsley.

PER SERVING: 100 calories; 5 g fat (45.2% calories from fat); 2 g protein; 13 g carbohydrate; 4 g dietary fiber; 0 mg cholesterol; 142 mg sodium. EXCHANGES: 1 vegetable; ½ fruit; 1 fat.

Mandarin Salad

Sesame oil and citrus provide an Asian tang.

MAKES 4 SERVINGS (8 CUPS)   PREPARATION TIME: 15 MINUTES

    1 tablespoon extra-virgin olive oil
    1 teaspoon sesame oil
    2 tablespoons lemon juice or rice wine vinegar
    1 teaspoon xylitol
    1 tablespoon low-sodium soy sauce
    4 cups fresh spinach, rinsed and dried
    2 cups lettuce (preferably romaine)
    ½ cup chopped celery
    2 green onions (with green tops), sliced
    1 cup (1 small can) mandarin oranges in water, chilled, drained,
       and patted dry
    ¼ cup sliced blanched almonds, for garnish

Prepare dressing by stirring together oils, lemon juice, xylitol, and soy sauce.

Tear spinach and lettuce into bite-sized pieces and mix in a large bowl with celery and green onions.

Just before serving, add oranges and dressing to greens and toss well. Top with almonds.

PER SERVING: 146 calories; 9 g fat (54.4% calories from fat); 4 g protein; 14 g carbohydrate; 3 g dietary fiber; 0 mg cholesterol; 197 mg sodium. EXCHANGES: ½ vegetable; ½ fruit; 1½ fat.

SERVING IDEA: Turn this into a main dish salad by topping with cooked, sliced chicken breast (half a breast or 4 ounces per serving).

Warm Spinach-Apple Salad

Much healthier than the usual version, which calls for bacon.

MAKES 4 SERVINGS (7 CUPS)   PREPARATION TIME: 15 MINUTES

6 cups fresh spinach, cleaned and dried
1 apple, cored and cut into ½-inch slices
2 tablespoons apple cider vinegar
2 tablespoons frozen apple juice concentrate
1 tablespoon extra-virgin olive oil
1 clove garlic, peeled and minced (optional)
¼ teaspoon Low-Sodium Seasoned Salt (page 297) or salt substitute
¼ cup pumpkin seeds, roasted

Place spinach in a large salad bowl, along with apple slices.

Combine apple cider vinegar, apple juice concentrate, olive oil, garlic, and salt in a small bowl and heat in a microwave for 30 to 45 seconds. (Or heat in a small saucepan over medium heat until hot, about 3 minutes.)

Pour hot dressing over salad, add pumpkin seeds, toss, and serve.

PER SERVING: 95 calories; 4 g fat (39.3% calories from fat); 2 g protein; 13 g carbohydrate; 3 g dietary fiber; 0 mg cholesterol; 124 mg sodium. EXCHANGES: ½ vegetable; ½ fruit; 1 fat.

Note
Pumpkin seeds, also known as *pepitas,* are a great source of zinc and health-enhancing omega-6 fatty acids.

Texas Caviar

Eat this on New Year's Day for good luck.

MAKES 3 SERVINGS (2 CUPS)   PREPARATION TIME: 12 HOURS

2 tablespoons extra-virgin olive oil
2 tablespoons red wine vinegar
1 clove garlic, peeled and minced
¼ teaspoon Low-Sodium Seasoned Salt (page 297)
    or salt substitute
¼ teaspoon freshly ground black pepper
¼ teaspoon garlic powder
¼ teaspoon onion powder
1 (15-ounce) can black-eyed peas, rinsed and drained
¼ cup finely chopped onion
¼ cup finely chopped green bell pepper
¼ cup finely chopped tomato

Combine olive oil, vinegar, garlic, and seasonings in a covered bowl and mix well.

Add black-eyed peas to the bowl along with onion, green pepper, and tomato. Stir well and refrigerate, at least overnight. (This will keep in the refrigerator for about a week.)

PER SERVING: 158 calories; 10 g fat (52.7% calories from fat); 4 g protein; 15 g carbohydrate; 3 g dietary fiber; 0 mg cholesterol; 355 mg sodium. EXCHANGES: ½ grain (starch); ½ lean meat; ½ vegetable; 2 fat.

Note
Tradition has it that if you eat black-eyed peas on New Year's Day, you'll have good luck—and plenty of pocket change—during the new year.

Tex-Mex Corn Salad

A perfect summer salad.

MAKES 4 SERVINGS (2 CUPS)   PREPARATION TIME: 40 MINUTES

¼ cup low-fat or fat-free mayonnaise

1 tablespoon skim milk

½ teaspoon chili powder

¼ teaspoon Low-Sodium Seasoned Salt (page 297) or salt substitute

¼ teaspoon freshly ground black pepper

2 cups corn, removed from cob or frozen, defrosted or canned, rinsed and drained

2 green onions (with green tops), thinly sliced

¼ cup diced celery

½ avocado, diced

1 tablespoon finely chopped parsley or cilantro

Combine mayonnaise, milk, chili powder, salt, and pepper in a small bowl, stir well.

In a large bowl, gently mix corn, green onions, celery, avocado, and dressing. Cover and chill for 30 minutes. Sprinkle parsley over salad before serving.

PER SERVING: 154 calories; 9 g fat (47.3% calories from fat); 3 g protein; 19 g carbohydrate; 3 g dietary fiber; 5 mg cholesterol; 184 mg sodium. EXCHANGES: 1 grain (starch); 1½ fat.

SERVING IDEA: This goes well with grilled poultry or fish.

Note

Corn has a moderately high glycemic index, but the ½-cup servings of this recipe shouldn't adversely affect your blood sugar.

Sweet Potato Salad

A decidedly different take on potato salad.

MAKES 6 SERVINGS (4 CUPS)   PREPARATION TIME: 2 HOURS

1 *pound (about 1½ large) sweet potatoes*
½ *cup chopped celery*
½ *cup chopped red bell peppers or green bell peppers*
3 *green onions (with green tops), chopped*
1 *tablespoon freshly chopped parsley*
¼ *cup low-fat or fat-free mayonnaise*
2 *tablespoons skim milk*
½ *teaspoon Low-Sodium Seasoned Salt (page 297) or salt substitute*
¼ *teaspoon freshly ground black pepper*
1½ *teaspoons Dijon mustard*

Scrub sweet potatoes, cut into quarters, and place in a medium saucepan. Cover with water, bring to a boil, then reduce heat and simmer for 15 to 20 minutes, until potatoes are just tender. Do not overcook—potatoes should be firm, not mushy. Drain, cool, and slip skins off. Cut potatoes into ½- to ¾-inch pieces and place in a medium bowl. Cool in refrigerator for at least 30 minutes.

Add celery, bell peppers, green onions, and parsley to potatoes and mix well.

Combine mayonnaise, milk, salt, pepper, and mustard and add to potatoes, stirring to coat well.

Cover and refrigerate for at least an hour, or overnight.

PER SERVING: 95 calories; 3 g fat (27.7% calories from fat); 1 g protein; 16 g carbohydrate; 2 g dietary fiber; 3 mg cholesterol; 197 mg sodium. EXCHANGES: 1 grain (starch); ½ vegetable; ½ fat.

(continued)

Sweet Potato Salad (continued)

Note

Sweet potatoes are loaded with beta-carotene and other protective carotenoids. Studies show that people who eat lots of carotenoid-rich fruits and vegetables are less likely to have heart disease, vision loss, and several types of cancer. Use the darker-skinned variety of sweet potatoes, which are also called yams, in this recipe.

Soups

Soup, glorious soup! It's comfort food, it's convenience food, it's hearty, healthy, stick-to-your-ribs food. We have provided an assortment of soups, from down-home (Grandma's Vegetable-Beefy Stew, page 157) to fancy (Cioppino, page 164) and everywhere in between. The recipes in this chapter provide you with the balance of protein, carbohydrate, and fat you need to keep blood sugar levels in balance. We've also tried to keep the sodium content in these recipes to a minimum—unlike canned and restaurant soups, which are overwhelmingly salty.

Because soup makes such wonderful leftovers—sometimes it tastes even better after the flavors blend in the fridge for a day or two—consider doubling or even tripling your favorite soup recipes. They will keep in the refrigerator for up to a week, and most soups freeze beautifully. We like to freeze extra soup in one- to two-cup containers that can be pulled out as needed. This is a great way to ensure healthy lunches that require only a quick reheat in the microwave.

The serving size for most of these recipes is 1¼ to 1½ cups. If you're having soup as your main course, plan for somewhat larger servings.

Ben's Chicken Noodle Soup

Thick, hearty, and filling

MAKES 6 SERVINGS (8 CUPS)   PREPARATION TIME: 30 MINUTES

2 *skinless, boneless chicken breast halves or 1–1½ cups diced
   cooked chicken*
7 *cups low-sodium chicken broth*
¼ *cup dry vermouth (optional)*
6 *ounces egg noodles*
½ *cup unbleached flour*
¾ *cup water*
1 *cup evaporated milk*
¼ *cup freshly chopped parsley*
⅛ *teaspoon freshly ground black pepper*

Place chicken, chicken broth, and vermouth in large saucepan or Dutch oven and bring to a boil. Reduce heat and simmer for about 10 to 15 minutes, until chicken is cooked. Remove chicken, cool slightly, and chop into bite-sized pieces. (If using cooked chicken, set aside until after noodles are cooked.)

Skim off any foam from stock, bring to rolling boil, and add noodles. Cook until just tender, about 10 minutes.

Meanwhile, stir flour into ¾ cup water and mix well. Slowly add to cooked noodles, along with evaporated milk, and stir as soup begins to thicken. Now add diced cooked chicken, and continue to cook, stirring constantly, for 2 more minutes, until soup is creamy.

Remove from heat, add chopped parsley and pepper, and stir well.

PER SERVING: 289 calories; 8 g fat (21.4% calories from fat); 30 g protein; 35 g carbohydrate; 1 g dietary fiber; 62 mg cholesterol;

128 mg sodium. EXCHANGES: 2 grain (starch); 2½ lean meat; ½ nonfat milk; ½ fat.

SERVING IDEA: For a hearty, informal dinner, serve this with Emerald Dip (page 62) and lots of raw veggies.

Chipotle Chili

Spicy, smoky, vegetarian and loaded with nutrients.

MAKES 6 SERVINGS (8 CUPS)

PREPARATION TIME:
1 HOUR 30 MINUTES (MINIMUM)

 1 teaspoon extra-virgin olive oil
 1 onion, chopped
 1 clove garlic, peeled and minced
 1 cup chopped celery
 1 cup chopped carrots
 1 cup chopped green bell pepper
 ½ cup ripe olives, sliced
 2 chipotle chiles canned in adobo sauce, chopped, plus a little
    sauce (more or less to taste—they're very hot) (see Note)
 1 (14½-ounce) can low-sodium tomatoes with juice, chopped
 ⅓ cup tomato paste
 1 (15-ounce) can kidney beans, rinsed and drained
 1 (12-ounce) bottle beer or 1½ cups water
1½ cups water
 2 tablespoons chili powder
 ½ teaspoon ground cumin

Heat olive oil in a large, heavy saucepan or Dutch oven over medium heat. Add onion, garlic, celery, carrots, and green pepper. Sauté for 10 minutes, stirring often.

Add olives, chiles, tomatoes, tomato paste, beans, beer, water, and spices. Stir well. Bring to a boil, reduce heat, and simmer for a minimum of 1 hour, stirring occasionally and adding more water, if necessary. Chili may be cooked for up to 4 hours, if you have the time. The longer you cook it, the better the flavor. In fact, chili is even better reheated the next day.

PER SERVING: 160 calories; 3 g fat (17% calories from fat); 7 g protein; 26 g carbohydrate; 8 g dietary fiber; 307 mg sodium. EXCHANGES: 1½ grain (starch); ½ lean meat; 2½ vegetable; ½ fat.

SERVING IDEAS: Top this with grated Cheddar cheese, nonfat or low-fat sour cream, chopped cilantro, or sliced green onions. You may also add ½ to 1 pound ground lean turkey to this recipe. Brown it along with the onions and other vegetables. Add extra water and seasonings to taste.

Note

Chipotle chiles are smoked, dried jalapeños that give food a spicy kick with smoky undertones. You can buy them dried, but the easiest way to use them is reconstituted in adobo sauce. Several manufacturers of Mexican foods make chipotle chiles canned in adobo sauce. If you can't find these in the ethnic section of your grocery store, substitute a small (3½-ounce) can of chopped green chiles and ¼ to ½ teaspoon red pepper flakes.

Tortilla Soup

Sopa de tortillas is always a crowd pleaser.

MAKES 8 SERVINGS (10 CUPS)   PREPARATION TIME: 1 HOUR

5 cups low-sodium chicken broth
2 cups water
2 skinless, boneless chicken breast halves, or 1 to 1½ cups diced cooked chicken
1 (14½-ounce) can low-sodium tomatoes with juice, chopped
1 medium onion, chopped
3 cloves garlic, peeled and minced
⅓ cup chopped cilantro
½ teaspoon cumin
2 chipotle chiles canned in adobo sauce, chopped, plus a little sauce (more or less to taste—they are very hot) (see Note, page 141)
1 cup coarsely crushed baked unsalted tortilla chips
¾ cup grated low-sodium Cheddar cheese or Monterey Jack cheese, for garnish
1 avocado, chopped, for garnish
2 limes, quartered

Place chicken broth, water, and chicken in a large saucepan or Dutch oven and bring to a boil. Reduce heat and simmer for 10 to 15 minutes, until chicken is cooked. Remove chicken, cool slightly, and chop into bite-sized pieces.

Skim off broth and add tomatoes with their juice, onion, garlic, cilantro, cumin, chiles, and diced chicken. Heat to boiling, reduce heat, and simmer for 30 minutes.

To serve, place 1 to 2 tablespoons of crushed tortilla chips in each of eight soup bowls and ladle soup over tortillas. Garnish each bowl with 1 tablespoon each cheese and avocado. Serve with lime wedges.

PER SERVING: 288 calories; 9 g fat (27.1% calories from fat); 21 g protein; 33 g carbohydrate; 4 g dietary fiber; 28 mg cholesterol; 386 mg sodium. EXCHANGES: 1½ grain (starch); 2 lean meat; ½ vegetable; 1½ fat.

Note

Avocados are at their best when they yield to gentle pressure. You can speed up the ripening of a hard avocado by placing it in a paper bag with an apple.

Rabbi Jake's Mushroom-Barley Soup

A hearty, homey soup that will stick to your ribs.

MAKES 6 SERVINGS (8 CUPS)   PREPARATION TIME: 1 HOUR 20 MINUTES

1 teaspoon extra-virgin olive oil
1 medium onion, chopped
2 stalks celery, chopped
1 large carrot, peeled and chopped
2 cloves garlic, minced
2 cups thinly sliced mushrooms
5 cups low-sodium beef, chicken, or vegetable broth
2 tablespoons low-sodium soy sauce
¾ cup pearl barley
1 teaspoon dried dill
2 tablespoons freshly chopped parsley

In a large, heavy saucepan or Dutch oven, heat olive oil over medium heat. Add onion, celery, carrot, and garlic and sauté, stirring occasionally, for 5 minutes. Add mushrooms and cook another minute.

Add broth, soy sauce, barley, dill, and parsley to the saucepan and bring to a boil. Reduce heat and simmer, stirring occasionally, for 50 to 60 minutes. Add ½ to 1 cup water if soup gets too thick.

PER SERVING: 162 calories; 1 g fat (6.5% calories from fat); 13 g protein; 26 g carbohydrate; 5 g dietary fiber; 0 mg cholesterol; 254 mg sodium. EXCHANGES: 1½ grain (starch); 1 lean meat; 1 vegetable.

Note
Barley may be even more effective than oats in controlling blood sugar and insulin levels, according to recent research.

Polish Sausage Stew

Kielbasa gives this hearty stew a nice, smoky flavor.

MAKES 8 SERVINGS (10 CUPS)   PREPARATION TIME: 1 HOUR

½ pound low-fat turkey kielbasa
4 cups low-sodium chicken broth
4 cups plus ½ to 1 cup water
1 onion, chopped
2 cloves garlic, peeled and minced
1 cup diced red potatoes (peeling optional)
1 (14½-ounce) can low-sodium tomatoes with juice, chopped, with juice reserved
½ cup cooked kidney beans, drained and rinsed, if canned
¼ teaspoon freshly ground black pepper
¼ teaspoon red pepper flakes
4 cups kale or other leafy greens (escarole, beet greens, spinach, etc.), cleaned, chopped, and loosely packed

Place turkey kielbasa in a medium saucepan and cover with water. Bring to a boil, reduce heat, and simmer for 10 minutes. Drain, cool, and chop.

Meanwhile, heat broth and 4 cups water in a large saucepan. Add onion, garlic, potatoes, tomatoes with their juice, beans, chopped sausage, and black pepper and red pepper flakes. Cook for 20 minutes, or until potatoes are tender. (If soup is very thick add an additional ½ to 1 cup water at this point.)

Add chopped kale to the saucepan and cook for 10 minutes, until tender. (If you're using spinach, you'll need to cook it only for 5 minutes or so.)

(continued)

Polish Sausage Stew *(continued)*

PER SERVING: 112 calories; 2 g fat (14.4% calories from fat); 13 g protein; 12 g carbohydrate; 2 g dietary fiber; 28 mg cholesterol; 533 mg sodium. EXCHANGES: ½ grain (starch); 1½ lean meat; 1½ vegetable.

SERVING IDEA: This is the way to eat fatty foods like sausage: buy turkey sausage, which is lower in fat, and use just enough to add flavor to your food.

Note

Leafy greens are nature's richest source of lutein and zeaxanthin, members of the carotenoid family that protect the eyes and particularly the retina from free radical damage. In a recent study, people who ate the most greens were least likely to develop macular degeneration, the leading cause of blindness in older people.

New Orleans Gumbo

A Louisiana specialty that can be made with chicken or seafood.

MAKES 6 SERVINGS (8 CUPS)   PREPARATION TIME: 55 MINUTES

¾ tablespoon *extra-virgin olive oil*
1 cup *chopped celery*
1 cup *chopped onion*
1 cup *chopped green bell pepper*
1 clove *garlic, peeled and minced*
¼ teaspoon *freshly ground black pepper*
¾ teaspoon *dried thyme*
4½ cups *low-sodium chicken broth*
1 (14½-ounce) can *low-sodium tomatoes with juice, chopped, with juice reserved*
1 *bay leaf*
2 cups *frozen okra, thawed and cut into ½-inch pieces*
1 cup *diced cooked chicken or whole small peeled shrimp*
½ cup *uncooked long-grain brown rice, rinsed*
Tabasco sauce (optional)

Heat olive oil over medium heat in a large, heavy saucepan or Dutch oven. Add celery, onion, green pepper, and garlic and cook, stirring often, until tender yet still crisp, 4 to 5 minutes. Stir in black pepper and thyme.

Add chicken broth to the saucepan, along with tomatoes with their juice, bay leaf, okra, chicken, and rice. Bring to a boil, then reduce heat, cover, and simmer for 30 to 35 minutes, until rice is tender. (If you use shrimp, add it during the final 10 minutes of cooking.)

Remove bay leaf and serve with Tabasco sauce.

(continued)

New Orleans Gumbo (*continued*)

PER SERVING: 188 calories; 3 g fat (16.1% calories from fat); 18 g protein; 22 g carbohydrate; 3 g dietary fiber; 20 mg cholesterol; 430 mg sodium. EXCHANGES: 1 grain (starch); 2 lean meat; 1½ vegetable; ½ fat.

Note

Gumbo comes from *gombo,* an African word for "okra," a signature ingredient in gumbo soups. If you don't have okra, use ½ teaspoon filé powder (ground sassafras leaves) as a thickener, adding it at the end, just before serving.

Minestrone Magnifico

Hearty, nutritious, Italian-inspired vegetable soup.

MAKES 6 SERVINGS (8 CUPS)   PREPARATION TIME: 50 MINUTES

½ tablespoon extra-virgin olive oil
¾ cup (about ½ medium) chopped onion
½ cup (about 1 small) chopped carrot
½ cup (about 1 stalk) chopped celery
2 cloves garlic, peeled and minced
1 cup (about 1 small) chopped zucchini
7 cups low-sodium chicken broth or vegetarian broth
½ (15-ounce) can cannellini beans or red kidney beans, rinsed
   and drained
2 tablespoons freshly chopped parsley
1 teaspoon Italian seasoning
⅛ teaspoon freshly ground black pepper
   Dash red pepper flakes
½ cup small pasta (fusilli, ditalini, or macaroni)
½ cup chopped cabbage
5 teaspoons grated Parmesan cheese

Heat olive oil in a large, heavy saucepan or Dutch oven over medium heat. Add onion, carrot, celery, and garlic and sauté for 3 minutes. Add zucchini and sauté for another 3 minutes.

Pour chicken broth into the saucepan, add beans, parsley, seasoning, black pepper, and red pepper flakes, and bring to a boil. Reduce heat and simmer for 20 minutes.

Add pasta and cabbage and simmer for 8 to 10 minutes. Cook until pasta is al dente, just barely tender. Add ½ to 1 cup water if soup is too thick.

(continued)

Minestrone Magnifico (continued)

Pour into six serving bowls and sprinkle each with 1 teaspoon cheese.

PER SERVING: 159 calories; 5 g fat (20.8% calories from fat); 19 g protein; 23 g carbohydrate; 4 g dietary fiber; 1 mg cholesterol; 87 mg sodium. EXCHANGES: 1 grain (starch); 2 lean meat; ½ vegetable; ½ fat.

SERVING IDEA: This is so hearty and wholesome, it is a meal in itself. Serve it with a salad.

Note

It seems as if every cookbook has its version of minestrone. This one is chock-full of vitamins and minerals. Make sure you add the cabbage at the very end. Cabbage's infamous odor, which is caused by sulfur compounds released during cooking, gets worse the longer you cook it, so limit cooking to 10 minutes.

Mexican Bean Chowder

Full of fiber and slow-burning carbohydrates.

MAKES 10 SERVINGS (12 CUPS)

PREPARATION TIME: 3 HOURS 15 MINUTES
(PLUS OVERNIGHT SOAKING)

1 *pound black beans*
1 *teaspoon extra-virgin olive oil*
1 *large onion, chopped*
4 *cloves garlic, peeled and minced*
8 *cups low-sodium chicken broth*
1 *large (7-ounce) can chopped green chiles, drained*
3 *tablespoons tomato paste*
¾ *cup freshly chopped cilantro*
¼ *teaspoon red pepper flakes, or to taste*
½ *cup Mary's Fresh Salsa (page 283) or Quick and Easy Salsa*
  (page 284) or store-bought low-sodium salsa
12 *teaspoons low-fat sour cream*
3 *limes, cut into fourths*

In a medium bowl or saucepan, cover beans with water and soak overnight. Before cooking, discard soaking water. Rinse beans thoroughly.

Heat olive oil in a large, heavy saucepan or Dutch oven over medium heat. Add onion and garlic and cook, stirring occasionally, for 4 to 5 minutes.

Pour broth into the saucepan and add beans, chiles, tomato paste, ½ cup cilantro, and pepper flakes. Bring to a boil, lower heat and skim off any foam that might rise to the surface. Simmer about 2 hours, until beans are soft. (Black beans remain firmer than most other beans. If you prefer more tender beans, add 1 to 2 cups water and cook for another hour.)

(continued)

Mexican Bean Chowder *(continued)*

To serve, ladle soup into eight bowls. Top each serving with 1 table-spoon salsa, 1 teaspoon sour cream (on top of salsa), and sprinkling of chopped cilantro. Serve with lime wedges.

PER SERVING (includes salsa): 237 calories; 1 g fat (6.0% calories from fat); 20 g protein; 38 g carbohydrate; 8 g dietary fiber; 1 mg cholesterol; 496 mg sodium. EXCHANGES: 2 grain (starch); 1½ lean meat; 1 vegetable.

SERVING IDEA: For a "dressier" soup, add 2 to 3 cups water and puree soup in blender. Do this 1 to 2 cups at a time and be careful not to burn yourself.

Note

Beans are an excellent source of soluble fiber, which lowers blood sugar in people with diabetes. Recent studies show that eating 50 grams of fiber a day lowers blood sugar by 10 percent.

Manhattan Clam Chowder

A nice change from creamy, fatty New England clam chowder.

MAKES 5 SERVINGS (6 CUPS)   PREPARATION TIME: 50 MINUTES

2 small (13-ounce) cans clams with juice (see Note)
2 cups low-sodium chicken broth plus more if needed
1 (14½-ounce) can low-sodium tomatoes, diced, with juice
1 medium onion, chopped
3 small new potatoes, chopped (peeling optional)
2 stalks celery, chopped
1 large carrot, chopped
1 clove garlic, peeled and minced
1 teaspoon Worcestershire sauce
½ teaspoon Low-Sodium Seasoned Salt (page 297) or salt substitute
¼ teaspoon freshly ground black pepper
½ teaspoon dried thyme or 1 heaping teaspoon freshly chopped
   thyme
4 teaspoons freshly chopped parsley, for garnish

Drain clams, reserving juice. Measure clam juice, then add enough broth to make 3 cups of liquid. Pour into a large saucepan.

Add tomatoes, onion, potatoes, celery, carrot, garlic, Worcestershire sauce, salt, pepper, and thyme to the saucepan. Bring to a boil over medium high heat, cover, lower heat, and simmer for 30 minutes, until potatoes are tender. (If soup is too thick at this point, add ½ to 1 cup water.)

Add clams to chowder, bring to a boil, and cook for 1 to 2 minutes. Ladle chowder into five bowls and garnish with chopped parsley.

(continued)

Manhattan Clam Chowder *(continued)*

PER SERVING: 224 calories; 2 g fat (7.5% calories from fat); 26 g protein; 26 g carbohydrate; 3 g dietary fiber; 49 mg cholesterol; 468 mg sodium. EXCHANGES: 1 grain (starch); 3 lean meat; 1½ vegetable.

SERVING IDEA: Serve this with a green salad and half a sandwich.

Note
If you want to use fresh clams, here's how to prepare them. Rinse about 2 dozen littleneck clams in a colander under cold water. Place in a large, covered saucepan or Dutch oven. Pour in ½ cup water, bring to a boil over high heat, reduce heat, and cook, shaking the saucepan occasionally, until the clams just open. This will take about 8 minutes. Throw out any clams that do not open.

Hot and Sour Soup

You won't believe how easy it is to make this
Chinese restaurant favorite.

MAKES 5 SERVINGS (5 CUPS)   PREPARATION TIME: 40 MINUTES

 8 dried shiitake mushrooms or dried wood ear mushrooms
 3½ cups low-sodium vegetable broth or chicken broth
 4 ounces white or brown mushrooms, cut into 1-inch matchsticks
    or julienned
 4 ounces extra-firm tofu, cut into 1-inch matchsticks
 ½ cup canned bamboo shoots, drained and cut into 1-inch
    matchsticks
 ¼ cup carrots, cut into 1-inch matchsticks
 3 tablespoons rice vinegar
 2 tablespoons low-sodium soy sauce
 2 teaspoons xylitol
 ¼ teaspoon freshly ground black pepper
 ¼ teaspoon red pepper flakes, or to taste
 2 tablespoons cornstarch
 3 tablespoons water
 1 egg white, lightly beaten
 1 teaspoon sesame oil
 2 green onions, thinly sliced

Soak dried shiitake mushrooms in very hot water for 30 minutes, until soft. Drain, cut off tough stems, and cut into thin slices.

In a large saucepan, bring broth, shiitakes, white mushrooms, tofu, bamboo shoots, and carrots to a boil. Reduce heat and simmer for 5 minutes.

(continued)

Hot and Sour Soup (continued)

Add vinegar, soy sauce, xylitol, black pepper, and red pepper flakes to the saucepan and cook for another minute.

Dissolve cornstarch in water and stir into soup. Stir constantly until soup begins to thicken. While stirring, slowly pour egg white into soup and cook until egg turns white.

Remove from heat and stir in sesame oil. Ladle into five serving bowls and top with green onions.

PER SERVING: 115 calories; 2 g fat (15.8% calories from fat); 12 g protein; 14 g carbohydrate; 4 g dietary fiber; 0 mg cholesterol; 621 mg sodium. EXCHANGES: ½ grain (starch); 1 lean meat; ½ vegetable; ½ fat.

SERVING IDEA: If you like your food hot and spicy, use hot sesame oil (also called chile oil).

Note

You'll find dried shiitake and wood ear mushrooms in Asian shops or the ethnic aisle of your supermarket. If you can't find them, don't worry—this recipe is delicious without them.

Grandma's Vegetable-Beefy Stew

This stew uses ground turkey in place of beef.

MAKES 6 SERVINGS (8 CUPS)   PREPARATION TIME: 1 HOUR 10 MINUTES

1 teaspoon extra-virgin olive oil
1 pound ground extra-lean turkey
2 cloves garlic
1 large onion, chopped
3 medium carrots, sliced ½ inch thick
3 stalks celery, sliced ½ inch thick
6 cups low-sodium beef broth
4 small new potatoes, diced (peeling optional)
1 (14½-ounce) can low-sodium tomatoes with juice, chopped, with juice reserved
2 teaspoons Worcestershire sauce
2 bay leaves
⅛ teaspoon red pepper flakes
½ teaspoon freshly ground black pepper
¼ teaspoon dried oregano
¼ teaspoon dried basil

Heat olive oil in a large, heavy saucepan or Dutch oven over medium heat. Add ground turkey and sauté, stirring frequently, until cooked through, 8 to 10 minutes.

Add garlic, onion, carrots, and celery to the saucepan and cook another 5 minutes, stirring occasionally.

Pour beef broth into the saucepan and add potatoes, tomatoes, Worcestershire sauce, bay leaves, and seasonings. Cook for 45 to 50 minutes, stirring occasionally and adding water to achieve desired consistency. Stew should be thick and hearty.

(continued)

Grandma's Vegetable-Beefy Stew *(continued)*

PER SERVING: 276 calories; 7 g fat (23.4% calories from fat); 27 g protein; 26 g carbohydrate; 4 g dietary fiber; 60 mg cholesterol; 170 mg sodium. EXCHANGES: 1 grain (starch); 3 lean meat; 1½ vegetable.

Note
You may also make this stew in a Crock-Pot. After browning turkey, place all ingredients in Crock-Pot and cook for 6 to 8 hours.

French Onion Soup

*Everybody loves French onion soup, and this recipe bypasses the
extreme saltiness that plagues many onion soups.*

MAKES 6 SERVINGS (8 CUPS)   PREPARATION TIME: 1 HOUR 25 MINUTES

2 tablespoon extra-virgin olive oil
7 cups (about 3 medium) thinly sliced onions
1 teaspoon xylitol
3 tablespoons unbleached flour
8 cups low-sodium beef broth
½ cup dry vermouth or dry white wine
2 tablespoons cognac (optional)
3 (½-inch) slices sourdough French bread, toasted and halved
2 ounces low-sodium Swiss cheese, grated

Heat olive oil in a large, heavy saucepan over medium heat. Add
onions and cook, stirring occasionally, for 5 minutes, or until soft.

Sprinkle xylitol over onions and continue to cook, stirring often,
for 30 minutes, until onions are golden brown. Reduce heat
slightly if onions brown too quickly.

Sprinkle flour over onions and cook, stirring for 2 minutes. Add
broth and vermouth to the saucepan, bring to a boil, then reduce
the heat and simmer over low heat for 30 minutes. Stir in cognac,
and remove from heat.

Preheat the broiler and arrange an oven shelf 5 to 6 inches from
heat source.

Ladle soup into six ovenproof serving bowls. Place slice of bread on
top of each bowl and sprinkle with grated cheese. Put the bowls on a
cookie sheet and place in oven for 1 to 2 minutes, until cheese melts.

(continued)

French Onion Soup *(continued)*

PER SERVING: 295 calories; 8 g fat (26% calories from fat); 21 g protein; 30 g carbohydrate; 4 g dietary fiber; 9 mg cholesterol; 140 mg sodium. EXCHANGES: ½ grain (starch); 2 lean meat; 3 vegetable; 1 fat.

Note

In addition to being low in calories and high in flavor, onions are one of our richest sources of quercetin. Quercetin acts as a potent antioxidant and has been proven to protect against cardiovascular disease by reducing blood clotting and guarding cholesterol against oxidation.

Easy Tortellini Soup

Try this with spinach, mushroom, or any other type of tortellini.

MAKES 4 SERVINGS (6 CUPS)   PREPARATION TIME: 25 MINUTES

3 cups low-sodium chicken broth
2 cups water
3 cloves garlic, peeled and minced, or more to taste
¼ teaspoon freshly ground black pepper
½ teaspoon Italian seasoning
6 ounces cheese-filled tortellini (fresh or frozen)
4 tightly packed cups (about 1 bunch) spinach, washed, stemmed, and chopped
¼ cup freshly chopped basil leaves, for garnish

Bring chicken broth, water, garlic, pepper, and seasoning to a boil in a medium saucepan.

Add tortellini and cook until just tender, 5 to 8 minutes for fresh tortellini and 10 plus minutes for frozen.

Add spinach and cook 2 to 3 minutes longer. Divide among four bowls and sprinkle with chopped basil.

PER SERVING: 164 calories; 3 g fat (14% calories from fat); 16 g protein; 20 g carbohydrate; 2 g dietary fiber; 29 mg cholesterol; 577 mg sodium. EXCHANGES: 1 grain (starch); 1½ lean meat; ½ vegetable; ½ fat.

SERVING IDEA: Throw together a hearty green salad and you can have dinner on the table in 30 minutes.

Note

In a pinch, you can use frozen chopped spinach, but fresh is much better in this recipe.

Curried Lentil Soup

Curry makes this version of lentil soup stand above the crowd.

MAKES 6 SERVINGS (6 CUPS)   PREPARATION TIME: 1 HOUR 5 MINUTES

1   teaspoon extra-virgin olive oil
1   large onion, chopped
3   cloves garlic, peeled and minced
2   teaspoons curry powder
⅛   teaspoon red pepper flakes, or to taste (they're very hot)
1   (14½-ounce) can low-sodium tomatoes, with juice
1   cup lentils, rinsed and drained
4   cups low-sodium chicken broth
½   cup freshly chopped cilantro, for garnish

Heat olive oil in a medium saucepan over medium heat. Add onion and garlic and cook 4 to 5 minutes, until soft. Add curry powder and red pepper flakes and cook, stirring for another minute.

Pour juice from tomatoes into the saucepan, then chop tomatoes and add to saucepan, along with lentils and broth. Bring to a boil, reduce heat, and simmer, stirring occasionally, for 40 to 50 minutes, until lentils are tender. (Add water, ½ cup at a time, if soup becomes too thick as it cooks.)

Pour into six serving bowls and top each with cilantro.

PER SERVING: 179 calories; 1 g fat (6.6% calories from fat); 18 g protein; 26 g carbohydrate; 11 g dietary fiber; 0 mg cholesterol; 362 mg sodium. EXCHANGES: 1½ grain (starch); 1½ lean meat; 1 vegetable.

Note

Lentils are the edible seeds of a member of the family of legumes, also called pulses. They are low in fat and high in fiber and provide an excellent source of protein. Traces of lentils have been found in five-thousand-year-old Mesopotamian settlements.

Cream of Broccoli Soup

Serve as a light first course to a formal meal.

MAKES 6 SERVINGS (6 CUPS)   PREPARATION TIME: 40 MINUTES

  1 teaspoon extra-virgin olive oil
  1 onion, chopped
  1 clove garlic, peeled and minced
  ½ teaspoon curry powder
  4 cups broccoli florets, coarsely chopped, or 1 16-ounce package
     frozen chopped broccoli, thawed and drained
1½ cups low-sodium chicken broth
  1 cup part-skim ricotta cheese
  1 cup evaporated skim milk
  ½ teaspoon Low-Sodium Seasoned Salt (page 297) or salt
     substitute
  ¼ teaspoon freshly ground black pepper

In a large saucepan, heat olive oil over medium heat. Add onion, garlic, and curry powder and cook, stirring often, for 3 to 4 minutes.

Add broccoli and broth to pan, bring to boil, and cook for 8 to 10 minutes until broccoli is tender. Add ricotta, milk, salt, and pepper.

Place soup in a food processor or blender and process just until smooth. (Unless your food processor or blender is very large, do half at a time.)

Return soup to the saucepan. Cook for 2 to 3 minutes over medium heat until hot, stirring often.

PER SERVING: 129 calories; 5 g fat (31.6% calories from fat); 11 g protein; 12 g carbohydrate; 2 g dietary fiber; 14 mg cholesterol; 358 mg sodium. EXCHANGES: ½ lean meat; 1 vegetable; ½ nonfat milk; ½ fat.

Cioppino

*Cioppino (chuh-PEE-no) is a robust, Italian-inspired fish stew
created in San Francisco.*

MAKES 6 SERVINGS (9 CUPS)   PREPARATION TIME: 1 HOUR 10 MINUTES

1 teaspoon extra-virgin olive oil
1 large onion, chopped
2 cloves garlic, peeled and minced
1 large green bell pepper, chopped
⅔ cup freshly chopped parsley
1 (28-ounce) can low-sodium tomatoes chopped with juice
1 (14½-ounce) can tomato sauce
1 cup clam juice
1 cup dry vermouth or dry white wine
1 bay leaf
1 teaspoon dried basil
1 teaspoon dried oregano
½ teaspoon freshly ground black pepper
¼ teaspoon red pepper flakes
12 clams or mussels, in their shells, scrubbed and ready for
    steaming
1 pound (20 to 25) large shrimp, shelled and deveined
¾ pound halibut fillets or other firm fish, cut into 1-inch pieces

Heat olive oil in a large, heavy saucepan or Dutch oven over
medium heat. Add onion, garlic, and green pepper and cook for
5 to 8 minutes until tender-crisp.

Stir in parsley, tomatoes, tomato sauce, clam juice, vermouth, bay
leaf, basil, oregano, black pepper, and red pepper flakes. Bring to a
boil, reduce heat, cover, and simmer for 15 minutes.

Add clams, shrimp, and halibut to the saucepan. Cover and simmer gently until clams pop open, shrimp turn pink, and fish is flaky, 10 to 15 minutes.

To serve, divide seafood among six bowls and ladle soup over top. Remove bay leaf before serving.

PER SERVING: 299 calories; 4 g fat (14% calories from fat); 34 g protein; 23 g carbohydrate; 4 g dietary fiber; 143 mg cholesterol; 759 mg sodium. EXCHANGES: 4½ lean meat; 2½ vegetable; ½ other carbohydrates.

SERVING IDEA: Cioppino is a meal in itself. Serve it with sourdough bread to mop up the sauce. (Limit bread to 1 slice per serving.)

Note
One way to simplify this recipe is to purchase precleaned fresh or frozen clams and shrimp. You may also include crab legs, mussels, and any other seafood of your choice.

Poultry

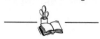

We love cooking poultry not only because it is a high-quality, low-fat source of protein, but also because it is so versatile. Chicken is equally delicious baked in a creamy sauce (Divine Chicken Divan, page 172), stir-fried in a wok (Almond Chicken Stir-Fry, page 183), and marinated and grilled (Jamaican Jerk Chicken, page 167). Turkey is also versatile, and you don't have to buy a twelve-pounder to enjoy it. Lean ground turkey and turkey bacon and sausage are good substitutes for their high-fat counterparts.

Check your supermarket or health food store for free-range poultry. You'll pay a little more, but you'll truly notice the difference in taste, and you'll rest assured that you're not getting the usual assortment of hormones and antibiotics fed to commercial livestock.

Many of the recipes in this section call for boneless, skinless chicken breast—it's the skin of the bird that contains most of its saturated fat. We suggest keeping bags of individually frozen chicken breasts in your freezer. Take out what you need and defrost it overnight or in the microwave. Just put a chicken breast, preferably marinated, under the broiler or on an outdoor grill or George Foreman grill, and your main course will be on the table inside of fifteen minutes. Nothing could be easier!

Jamaican Jerk Chicken
Hot and spicy.

MAKES 6 SERVINGS   PREPARATION TIME: 3 HOURS

1 *bunch green onions, coarsely chopped*
3 *cloves garlic, peeled*
1 *small serrano or jalapeño chile, to taste*
2 *tablespoons lemon juice*
2 *tablespoons lime juice*
2 *tablespoons freshly chopped thyme or 1 teaspoon dried thyme*
1 *tablespoon extra-virgin olive oil*
1 *tablespoon freshly ground black pepper*
1 *tablespoon freshly ground coriander seeds or 1 teaspoon dried coriander*
1 *bay leaf*
¼ *teaspoon salt or salt substitute*
1 *(4-pound) broiler or fryer chicken or 4 pounds thighs, legs, or breasts*
   Olive oil spray
4 *lime wedges*

Make jerk rub by combining all except last 3 ingredients in a food processor or blender and process until thick paste forms. (Be careful when handling chiles.) Set aside.

Rinse chicken and remove skin and excess fat. Split in half lengthwise and place in a shallow glass pan. Reserve ¼ cup jerk rub and rub rest into all surfaces of chicken. Cover and refrigerate at least 2 hours, turning occasionally.

Preheat a grill to medium high (350 to 400 degrees F) and spray the rack with olive oil spray. (Or preheat the broiler and spray the broiler pan.)

(continued)

Jamaican Jerk Chicken *(continued)*

Cook chicken on the grill, turning occasionally and basting with reserved jerk rub. Cook until firm and juices run clear when chicken is pricked with a fork. (If you're using chicken pieces with bones, total cooking time will be about 30 to 40 minutes. If you use boneless chicken breasts, cooking time will be about 7 minutes per side.)

Serve hot, with lime wedges.

PER SERVING: 239 calories; 9 g fat (34.9% calories from fat); 34 g protein; 4 g carbohydrate; 1 g dietary fiber; 143 mg cholesterol; 239 mg sodium. EXCHANGES: 5 lean meat; ½ fat.

SERVING IDEA: Try this with Sweet Potato Salad (page 135).

Note
"Jerking" meat is a Jamaican tradition, initially used to mask the strong flavor of wild boar. It involves rubbing citrus juice, peppers, and spice into the meat and marinating before cooking. Jerk marinade is very hot. If you prefer your food less spicy, cut back on chiles and black peppers; if you're a real fireball, add more.

Elegant Roasted Chicken

A dish that should be in every cook's repertoire.

MAKES 8 SERVINGS   PREPARATION TIME: 2 HOURS

1   (6-pound) roasting chicken
1   teaspoon extra-virgin olive oil
½   teaspoon salt or salt substitute
½   teaspoon freshly ground black pepper

Preheat the oven to 425 degrees F. Place a rack in a roasting pan or medium baking dish.

Remove giblets and extra fat, rinse chicken well inside and out, and dry with paper towels. Rub olive oil all over chicken and sprinkle with salt and pepper. Place in the prepared pan, breast side up.

Cook 1 hour and 15 to 30 minutes, or until thermometer inserted in the breast or thigh reads 170 degrees F. Basting isn't necessary, although you may baste occasionally with pan drippings if you wish. If the drippings begin to smoke, remove them with a spoon or baster, and add 2 or 3 tablespoons of water to the bottom of the pan.

Drain juices from the cavity of the chicken and let sit for 10 to 15 minutes before serving.

PER SERVING (includes skin, see Note): 428 calories; 32 g fat (67.8% calories from fat); 34 g protein; trace carbohydrate; trace dietary fiber; 143 mg cholesterol; 240 mg sodium. EXCHANGES: 1 grain (starch); 4½ lean meat; 3½ fat.

(continued)

Elegant Roasted Chicken (continued)

SERVING IDEA: Roasted chicken goes well with almost anything, and it's good hot or cold. A 6-pound chicken may sound like a lot, but the 6- to 8-pound roasters have the best flavor. Use leftover chicken for sandwiches or dishes such as Divine Chicken Divan (page 172).

Note

It is important that you remove the skin before eating to dramatically cut back on fat and calories. Nutritional analysis above is with skin. If you remove the skin, the fat content drops down to about 8 grams and the calories to less than 200.

Easy Baked Barbecue Chicken
Only four ingredients and no fuss.

MAKES 4 SERVINGS   PREPARATION TIME: 1 HOUR

Olive oil spray
4 *(4-ounce) skinless, boneless chicken breast halves*
1 *medium onion, thinly sliced*
1 *medium green bell pepper, chopped*
¾ *cup barbecue sauce (see Note)*

Preheat the oven to 350 degrees F. Spray the bottom of an 8-by-8-inch baking pan with olive oil spray.

Place chicken in the prepared pan. Sprinkle onion and green pepper over chicken and pour barbecue sauce evenly over top.

Cover and bake for 30 to 40 minutes. Remove cover and continue baking 10 minutes, or until chicken is firm and juices run clear.

PER SERVING: 178 calories; 2 g fat (12.2% calories from fat); 28 g protein; 10 g carbohydrate; 2 g dietary fiber; 66 mg cholesterol; 457 mg sodium. EXCHANGES: 3½ lean meat; ½ vegetable; ½ other carbohydrates.

SERVING IDEA: This goes well with 21st-Century Waldorf Salad (page 123).

Note
Look for low-sodium barbecue sauce to reduce the sodium content of this recipe.

Divine Chicken Divan

Chicken Divan is named for its place of origin, the Divan Parisien,
a New York City restaurant popular in the 1950s.

MAKES 6 SERVINGS   PREPARATION TIME: 1 HOUR 10 MINUTES

1   *pound boneless, skinless chicken breast or 2½ cups cooked*
    chicken or turkey

1½ *pounds broccoli spears, trimmed, or 2 (10-ounce) packages*
    frozen broccoli spears, thawed
    Olive oil spray

1½ *cups skim milk*

1   *(10¾-ounce) can condensed, reduced-fat, reduced-sodium*
    cream of mushroom soup

2   *tablespoons dry sherry*

⅛   *teaspoon ground nutmeg*

½   *teaspoon curry powder*

¼   *teaspoon freshly ground black pepper*

3   *tablespoons whole wheat flour*

½   *cup grated low-sodium Cheddar cheese*

½   *cup grated Parmesan cheese*

Cut chicken breast into 3 or 4 pieces. Place chicken in a large saucepan, cover with water, and bring to a boil. Cook for about 10 minutes until cooked through. Remove, cool, and cut into bite-sized pieces. If you're using cooked chicken or turkey simply cut into bite-sized pieces. (This is a great way to use leftovers.)

Meanwhile, steam broccoli spears. Place in a microwave-proof dish, add 2 tablespoons of water, cover, and cook for 2 to 3 minutes, until tender but crisp. (May also be cooked in a steamer for a few minutes.)

Preheat the oven to 350 degrees F. Prepare an 8-by-8-inch baking pan by spraying with olive oil spray.

Place 1¼ cups milk, cream of mushroom soup, sherry, and spices in a medium saucepan. In a small bowl, stir flour into remaining ¼ cup milk and mix well. Pour into the saucepan. Bring to a boil over medium heat, stirring constantly with a wire whisk. Cook for about 8 minutes, until the sauce is thick and creamy.

Place broccoli spears in prepared baking pan. Layer chicken on top of broccoli. Sprinkle Cheddar cheese evenly over chicken. Pour sauce over top. Cover and bake for 20 minutes. Remove cover, sprinkle with Parmesan cheese, and continue cooking for 15 minutes, until hot and bubbly.

If desired, place under a preheated broiler for about 2 to 3 minutes, until top is lightly browned.

PER SERVING: 246 calories; 8 g fat (28.9% calories from fat); 28 g protein; 15 g carbohydrate; 3 g dietary fiber; 62 mg cholesterol; 456 mg sodium. EXCHANGES: ½ grain (starch); 3 lean meat; ½ vegetable; 1 fat.

SERVING IDEA: Round out this meal with a salad, such as Warm Spinach-Apple Salad (page 132).

Note
This is a lighter version of the original Chicken Divan, which was made with Mornay sauce (cheese, butter, and milk). An apology to purists who shun canned soups, but the only way we could come close to duplicating this divine recipe without all the saturated fat was with reduced-fat cream of mushroom soup.

Crispy Chicken Tenders

If you like Chicken McNuggets, you'll love these.

MAKES 4 SERVINGS   PREPARATION TIME: 30 MINUTES

Olive oil spray
1   pound skinless, boneless chicken breast
2   large egg whites or ¼ cup Egg Beaters or other egg white product
½   tablespoon water
¼   cup unbleached flour
½   teaspoon Low-Sodium Seasoned Salt (page 297) or salt substitute
½   cup bread crumbs (preferably sprouted-grain)

Preheat the oven to 400 degrees F. Spray a nonstick cookie sheet or jelly roll pan with olive oil spray.

Cut chicken lengthwise into 1-by-4-inch strips.

In a shallow bowl, whisk egg whites with water until foamy.

Mix flour with salt and spread out on a plate. Place bread crumbs on a second plate. Dip chicken strips, one at a time, in flour, then in egg white, then in bread crumbs, turning to coat both sides.

Place chicken on the prepared cookie sheet. Bake for 6 minutes, turn, and bake another 6 to 8 minutes, or until golden brown and tender.

PER SERVING: 213 calories; 2 g fat (10.0% calories from fat); 31 g protein; 15 g carbohydrate; 1 g dietary fiber; 66 mg cholesterol; 389 mg sodium. EXCHANGES: 1 grain (starch); 4 lean meat.

SERVING IDEA: Serve this with a variety of prepared dipping sauces: Mandarin Dipping Sauce (page 291), Farm Dressing and Dip (page 276), barbecue sauce, or ketchup.

Coq au Vin

A trimmed-down version of a popular French dish.

MAKES 8 SERVINGS   PREPARATION TIME: 1 HOUR 15 MINUTES

  1 teaspoon paprika
 ½ teaspoon Low-Sodium Seasoned Salt (page 297) or salt substitute
 ½ teaspoon freshly ground black pepper
  3 large chicken thighs, skin removed
  3 large chicken legs, skin removed
  1 large boneless, skinless chicken breast
  4 teaspoons extra-virgin olive oil
  2 large onions, sliced
  1 large carrot, sliced
  2 stalks celery, sliced
  2 cloves garlic, peeled and chopped
  3 tablespoons unbleached flour
  2 tablespoons brandy (optional)
  2 cups red wine (zinfandel, Mâcon, or Chianti)
  2 cups low-sodium chicken broth
  3 sprigs fresh thyme or 1 teaspoon dried thyme
  3 bay leaves
 16 ounces mushrooms (preferably whole small; if large, halved or
     quartered)
 12 shallots, peeled

Combine seasonings in a small bowl. Rub over all surfaces of
chicken pieces.

Heat 1 teaspoon olive oil in a large heavy Dutch oven or skillet over
medium heat. Add chicken pieces in a single layer and brown, 3 to
5 minutes on each side. Repeat with remaining chicken pieces,
adding another teaspoon of oil. Remove from the Dutch oven.

(continued)

Coq au Vin (continued)

Add another teaspoon of olive oil to the Dutch oven. Place the onions, carrot, celery, and garlic in the Dutch oven and cook, stirring frequently, for 5 minutes, until onions begin to turn translucent.

Stir in flour and cook, stirring, for an additional minute. Pour in brandy, wine, and chicken broth, and add thyme and bay leaves. Bring to a boil. Spoon liquid over chicken pieces—they should be barely covered with liquid. Reduce heat to a simmer, loosely covered (place lid ajar so it is not completely sealed). Cook for 15 minutes, then turn chicken.

Meanwhile, heat final teaspoon of olive oil in a large nonstick skillet over medium-high heat. Add mushrooms and shallots and cook, stirring often, until browned, about 5 minutes. Add to pot after chicken has cooked 15 minutes. Stir gently.

Continue cooking. Total cooking time will be 25 to 35 minutes, depending on your bird. Chicken is done when it is cooked through and tender, yet not falling off the bone.

When it is done, remove chicken, bring sauce to a boil, and cook for 5 minutes or so, until sauce is reduced a bit. (It will still be thin.) Return chicken to pot, cook for a minute or two, and serve.

PER SERVING: 259 calories; 6 g fat (24.8% calories from fat); 27 g protein; 13 g carbohydrate; 2 g dietary fiber; 78 mg cholesterol; 354 mg sodium. EXCHANGES: 3½ lean meat; 1½ vegetable; ½ fat.

SERVING IDEAS: Serve this with Quinoa Pilaf (page 268), a green salad, and a nice red wine. Coq au Vin is even better after it's sat in the fridge for a day or two.

Chicken Paprika

A delicious, light version of a Hungarian classic.

MAKES 4 SERVINGS   PREPARATION TIME: 1 HOUR

2   teaspoons extra-virgin olive oil
2   cups chopped onions
1   clove garlic, minced
1½ cups mushrooms, sliced
4   (4-ounce) boneless, skinless chicken breast halves
2   tablespoons lemon juice
2   teaspoons paprika (preferably Hungarian)
½   teaspoon salt or salt substitute
¼   teaspoon freshly ground black pepper
4   ounces egg noodles
1   tablespoon unbleached flour
⅔   cup skim milk
½   cup low-fat sour cream

Heat 1 teaspoon olive oil in a large nonstick skillet over medium heat. Add onions and garlic and cook for 3 minutes, stirring often. Add mushrooms and cook another minute or two. Remove from the skillet.

Add remaining teaspoon of olive oil, heat, and then add chicken. Brown lightly, cooking for about 3 minutes on each side. Sprinkle lemon juice, paprika, salt, and pepper over chicken. Return onions and mushrooms to skillet with chicken, reduce heat, and cover tightly. Cook over low heat until chicken is tender, 12 to 15 minutes. Remove chicken from skillet and keep warm.

(continued)

Chicken Paprika (continued)

While chicken is cooking (time it so they'll be done at the same time the chicken dish is done), cook egg noodles per package instructions. (Or bring 6 cups of water to a rapid boil, add noodles, and cook 8 to 9 minutes until al dente.) Drain.

Turn heat up to medium. Sprinkle flour over onions and mushrooms and cook, stirring constantly, for 1 minute. Pour in milk and simmer, stirring often, until thickened, about 3 minutes. Stir in sour cream. Add chicken and cook until heated through, but do not boil.

Serve over egg noodles.

PER SERVING: 359 calories; 7 g fat (17.3% calories from fat); 36 g protein; 37 g carbohydrate; 3 g dietary fiber; 102 mg cholesterol; 275 mg sodium. EXCHANGES: 1½ grain (starch); 4 lean meat; 1½ vegetable; 1 fat.

SERVING IDEA: All you need for a complete meal is a green salad. Try this with Warm Spinach-Apple Salad (page 132).

Note
Vitamin C was first isolated from ripe paprika pods by Hungarian chemist Albert Szent-Györgyi, who went on to win the Nobel Prize in 1937 for this work.

Chicken Jambalaya

A lighter version of a famous New Orleans dish.

MAKES 4 SERVINGS   PREPARATION TIME: 1 HOUR

- 2 teaspoons extra-virgin olive oil
- 4 ounces low-fat chicken andouille, kielbasa, or other low-fat smoked turkey or chicken sausage, cut into bite-sized pieces
- 8 ounces (2 breast halves) boneless, skinless chicken breast, cut into ½-inch cubes
- 1 small onion, chopped
- 3 stalks celery, chopped
- ½ green bell pepper, chopped
- 3 cloves garlic, peeled and minced
- 1 (14½-ounce) can low-sodium tomatoes with juice
- 1½ cups low-sodium chicken broth
- ⅔ cup long-grain brown rice
- 1 bay leaf
- ½ teaspoon dried oregano
- ½ teaspoon freshly ground black pepper
- ½ teaspoon dried thyme
- ¼ teaspoon cayenne pepper
- ¼ teaspoon Tabasco sauce, or to taste

Heat 1 teaspoon olive oil in a large, heavy covered skillet or Dutch oven over medium heat. Add sausage and chicken and cook for 4 to 5 minutes, stirring often, until chicken is cooked through. Remove and set aside.

Add second teaspoon of olive oil, along with onion, celery, green pepper, and garlic to skillet. Cook, stirring occasionally, until tender-crisp, about 5 minutes. (Add a couple of tablespoons of water if onions stick or begin to burn.)

(continued)

Chicken Jambalaya (continued)

Return sausage and chicken to skillet and add tomatoes with their juice, chicken broth, rice, spices, and Tabasco sauce. Bring to a boil, reduce heat, cover, and simmer for 35 to 45 minutes until rice is tender. Fluff with a fork, correct spices (add more cayenne or Tabasco if desired), remove bay leaf, and serve.

PER SERVING: 295 calories; 6 g fat (17.7% calories from fat); 26 g protein; 35 g carbohydrate; 4 g dietary fiber; 61 mg cholesterol; 524 mg sodium. EXCHANGES: 1½ grain (starch); 3 lean meat; 2 vegetable; ½ fat.

SERVING IDEA: There are dozens of ways to make jambalaya, without tomatoes (Cajun-style brown jambalaya), with shrimp—even with alligator. This one-pot recipe can be doubled to feed a crowd.

Chicken Fajitas

Equally good with chicken or shrimp.

MAKES 4 SERVINGS   PREPARATION TIME: 1 HOUR 20 MINUTES

¼ cup lime juice

2 cloves garlic, peeled and minced

1 teaspoon ground coriander

1 teaspoon ground cumin

¼ teaspoon red pepper flakes

½ pound boneless, skinless chicken breast, cut into 1½-by-1-inch strips

4 whole wheat tortillas

Olive oil spray

1 large green bell pepper or mixture of red and green bell peppers, sliced lengthwise

1 medium onion, sliced lengthwise, plus ½ cup chopped onion

1 cup chopped tomatoes

1 cup shredded lettuce

½ cup grated low-sodium Cheddar cheese

½ cup Mary's Fresh Salsa (page 283) or Quick and Easy Salsa (page 284) or store-bought low-sodium salsa

½ cup Guacamole (page 55) (optional)

Combine lime juice, garlic, coriander, cumin, and pepper flakes in a large bowl. Stir to mix well.

Add chicken strips to the bowl and stir to completely coat with marinade. Cover and refrigerate for at least 1 hour.

To prepare tortillas, heat a large nonstick skillet over medium heat. Place tortillas, one at a time, in the skillet and heat 30 seconds to 1 minute on each side until pliable and warm. Keep warm.

(continued)

Chicken Fajitas (continued)

Heat a large nonstick skillet over medium-high heat. Spray with olive oil spray.

Add chicken to the skillet and cook, stirring frequently, for 3 to 4 minutes until done. Remove from the skillet.

Add green pepper and sliced onion to the skillet and stir-fry until tender-crisp, about 5 minutes. Return chicken to the skillet and cook a minute or two until heated through.

Spoon one-fourth of the chicken-vegetable mixture onto each tortilla. Top with tomatoes, lettuce, chopped onion, cheese, and a spoonful each of salsa and guacamole.

PER SERVING (includes salsa and guacamole): 291 calories; 11 g fat (29.4% calories from fat); 22 g protein; 35 g carbohydrate; 4 g dietary fiber; 47 mg cholesterol; 398 mg sodium. EXCHANGES: 1½ grain (starch); 2½ lean meat; 2 vegetable; 1½ fat.

SERVING IDEA: Half a pound of cleaned, peeled shrimp may be used in place of chicken.

Note
A tortilla warmer is a good investment if you cook Mexican food often. It keeps tortillas warm and prevents them from drying out.

Almond Chicken Stir-Fry

Almonds give this a nice crunch!

MAKES 4 SERVINGS   PREPARATION TIME: 45 MINUTES

½ pound (2 breast halves) boneless, skinless chicken breast
2 tablespoons low-sodium soy sauce
¾ cup long-grain brown rice
1½ cups water
½ cup low-sodium chicken or vegetable broth
1 clove garlic, peeled and minced
1 teaspoon grated gingerroot or ¼ teaspoon ground ginger
   Dash red pepper flakes
1 tablespoon cornstarch
   Olive oil spray
1 teaspoon extra-virgin olive oil
1 onion, halved and thinly sliced lengthwise
1 green bell pepper, thinly sliced into 1-inch lengths
1 carrot, peeled and cut into 1-inch matchsticks
1 small zucchini, cut into 1-inch matchsticks
⅓ cup almonds

Cut chicken into ¼ inch by 1 inch pieces. (This is much easier with partially frozen chicken. If yours is defrosted, place in freezer for 30 minutes before slicing.) Place in a small bowl and toss with 1 tablespoon soy sauce. Refrigerate.

Prepare rice per package directions. (Rinse, cover with water, bring to a boil and simmer 35 to 45 minutes, until soft and water has evaporated.)

Meanwhile, mix broth, 1 tablespoon soy sauce, garlic, ginger, and red pepper flakes in a small bowl. Stir in cornstarch.

(continued)

Almond Chicken Stir-Fry *(continued)*

Heat a large nonstick wok or skillet over medium-high heat and spray with olive oil spray. Add chicken and cook, stirring often, until chicken is done, about 3 minutes. Remove from the wok and keep warm.

Add onion slices, green pepper, carrot and zucchini to the wok and cook, stirring often, for 3 to 4 minutes, until tender-crisp.

Return chicken to the wok and cook for 1 minute. Add sauce and stir constantly for 1 to 2 minutes as sauce thickens.

Stir in almonds and serve over brown rice.

PER SERVING: 309 calories; 8 g fat (23.1% calories from fat); 21 g protein; 40 g carbohydrate; 5 g dietary fiber; 33 mg cholesterol; 358 mg sodium. EXCHANGES: 2 grain (starch); 2 lean meat; 1½ vegetable; 1½ fat.

SERVING IDEA: Round out this meal with a green salad. Try Island Breeze Salad (page 126) or Orange County Special (page 130).

Turkey Tetrazzini
A light version of a magnificent dish.

8 *ounces spaghetti*
1 *teaspoon extra-virgin olive oil*
8 *ounces mushrooms (preferably small whole; if large, halved or quartered)*
   Olive oil spray
1½ *cups low-sodium chicken broth*
¼ *cup dry sherry*
¾ *cup evaporated skim milk*
2 *tablespoons cornstarch*
2 *cups cooked turkey or chicken, cut into 1-inch pieces*
¼ *teaspoon salt or salt substitute*
⅛ *teaspoon freshly ground black pepper*
½ *cup grated low-sodium Cheddar cheese*
2 *tablespoons grated Parmesan cheese*

Cook spaghetti in boiling water per package directions. Drain and rinse. Return to the cooking pot.

Meanwhile, heat olive oil in a large nonstick skillet over medium heat. Add mushrooms and cook, stirring often, until lightly browned, about 5 minutes.

Preheat the oven to 350 degrees F. Spray a 9-by-13-inch baking pan with olive oil spray.

In a large saucepan, combine broth and sherry, and bring to a boil over medium heat. Reduce heat and simmer for 5 minutes.

(continued)

Turkey Tetrazzini (continued)

In a small bowl, stir milk and cornstarch together until cornstarch dissolves. Slowly pour into broth, stirring constantly as it returns to a boil and thickens. Reduce heat and simmer for 3 minutes. Sauce should be thick and creamy. Add turkey and mushrooms to sauce and cook, stirring, for 1 minute.

Pour sauce over cooked pasta, stir to mix well, then transfer to the prepared baking pan. Add salt and pepper, and sprinkle Cheddar and Parmesan cheese over top. Cover.

Bake for 20 minutes. Remove cover and bake another 10 minutes until golden brown and bubbly.

PER SERVING: 352 calories; 9 g fat (26.9% calories from fat); 27 g protein; 36 g carbohydrate; 1 g dietary fiber; 55 mg cholesterol; 203 mg sodium. EXCHANGES: 2 grain (starch); 2½ lean meat; ½ vegetable; 1 fat.

SERVING IDEA: Serve this with a hearty, vegetable-dense salad such as Luscious Layered Salad (page 120).

Note

This dish was created almost a century ago for Italian soprano Luisa Tetrazzini. The original dish included chicken and lots of cream, as befitting the Rubenesque diva. This lighter version is delicious—and a great way to use leftover turkey.

Two-Hour Roasted Turkey

Who says you have to save turkey with all the fixings for holidays?
Try this hassle-free recipe any time of the year.

MAKES 12 SERVINGS   PREPARATION TIME: 2½ HOURS

4 pounds turkey breast (whole breast, sometimes called turkey
  roast)
1 teaspoon extra-virgin olive oil
¼ teaspoon Low-Sodium Seasoned Salt (page 297) or salt substitute
¼ teaspoon freshly ground black pepper

Preheat the oven to 325 degrees F.

Rub turkey with olive oil, salt, and pepper and place on a rack in a
roasting pan or in a shallow baking pan. Place a meat thermometer
in turkey, making sure it doesn't touch a bone.

Bake until the thermometer registers 170 degrees F, about 2 hours.
If turkey begins to get too brown, cover loosely with aluminum foil.

Let sit for 10 minutes, remove skin, and carve.

PER SERVING: 217 calories; 10 g fat (42.8% calories from fat); 30 g
protein; trace carbohydrate; trace dietary fiber; 89 mg cholesterol;
109 mg sodium. EXCHANGE: 4 lean meat.

SERVING IDEAS: Don't forget to remove the skin before serving—
that's where the bulk of the saturated fat resides. Serve with Pecan
Stuffing (page 269), Gravy (page 293), and Fresh Cranberry-Orange
Relish (page 295).

Note

Whole turkey breasts (bone in, skin on) and turkey roasts (usually
boned and skinned) take the fuss out of cooking turkey. They're
also great for smaller crowds and white meat lovers.

Ginger-Soy Chicken Breasts

Teriyaki-style chicken that's a snap to prepare.

MAKES 4 SERVINGS   PREPARATION TIME: 2½ HOURS

¼ cup low-sodium soy sauce
¼ cup water
2 tablespoons rice wine or dry sherry
1 teaspoon grated gingerroot or ½ teaspoon ground ginger
1 clove garlic, peeled and minced
4 (4-ounce) skinless, boneless chicken breast halves
   Olive oil spray

Combine soy sauce, water, rice wine, ginger, and garlic in a small bowl. Heat in a microwave for 3 minutes, or boil in a small saucepan for 3 minutes. Cool.

Place chicken in a tightly sealed container or plastic bag and pour sauce over it. Seal and turn to coat chicken pieces evenly. Marinate in the refrigerator at least 2 hours or overnight, turning occasionally.

Preheat a grill, broiler, or George Foreman grill. Spray it with olive oil spray.

Place chicken on the grill, brush with marinade, and cook 7 to 9 minutes on each side, turning once. If you're using a George Foreman grill, total cooking time will be about 5 minutes, depending on thickness.

PER SERVING: 146 calories; 1 g fat (9.8% calories from fat); 27 g protein; 2 g carbohydrate; trace dietary fiber; 66 mg cholesterol; 674 mg sodium. EXCHANGES: 3½ lean meat; ½ vegetable.

Skillet Supper

A hearty and easy one-dish meal.

MAKES 6 SERVINGS   PREPARATION TIME: 40 MINUTES

4 *ounces elbow macaroni*
Olive oil spray
1 *pound lean ground turkey*
1 *large onion, chopped*
1 *large green bell pepper, chopped*
2 *cloves garlic, peeled and minced*
1 *(14½-ounce) can low-sodium tomatoes with juice, chopped*
¾ *cup low-sodium V8 juice or tomato sauce*
1 *teaspoon paprika*
¼ *teaspoon salt or salt substitute*
¼ *teaspoon freshly ground black pepper*
½ *cup low-fat sour cream*

Cook macaroni in rapidly boiling water just until tender, about 7 minutes, per package instructions. Drain, rinse, and set aside.

Meanwhile, spray a large nonstick skillet with olive oil spray. Heat over medium heat and add turkey. Cook, stirring occasionally and breaking up with wooden spoon until meat begins to brown, about 8 minutes.

Add onion, green pepper, and garlic to the skillet and continue cooking for another 5 minutes. Add tomatoes, V8 juice, paprika, salt, pepper, and macaroni. Bring to a boil, then reduce heat to a simmer. Cover and cook for 10 minutes.

Remove lid, turn up heat, and cook for 5 minutes or so, until most of the liquid evaporates. (It should be juicy, rather than completely dry.) Stir in sour cream, heat for another minute, and serve.

(continued)

Skillet Supper *(continued)*

PER SERVING: 237 calories; 77 g fat (25.6% calories from fat); 20 g protein; 24 g carbohydrate; 2 g dietary fiber; 54 mg cholesterol; 182 mg sodium. EXCHANGES: 1 grain (starch); 2 lean meat; 1½ vegetable.

SERVING IDEA: All you need is a green salad for a complete meal. Try Blue Cheese Lovers' Salad (page 125) or Warm Spinach-Apple Salad (page 132).

Note

Use the leanest ground turkey you can find. Regular ground turkey contains quite a bit of fat, since it's ground with skin. The leanest of all is ground turkey breast.

Pecan-Crusted Chicken
Crunchy and delicious.

MAKES 4 SERVINGS PREPARATION TIME: 4 HOURS 40 MINUTES

1 cup nonfat plain yogurt
1 tablespoon lemon juice
4 (4-ounce) skinless, boneless chicken breast halves
Olive oil spray
2 cups Kellogg's Special K cereal
⅓ cup finely chopped pecans
½ teaspoon seasoned salt or salt substitute
1 teaspoon lemon pepper

Combine yogurt and lemon juice in a small bowl.

Rinse and dry chicken. Cut into 4 pieces.

Place chicken in a shallow baking dish and cover with yogurt mixture, turning to coat evenly. Cover and refrigerate for at least 4 hours, or overnight, turning occasionally.

Preheat the oven to 450 degrees F. Spray a nonstick baking sheet or jelly roll pan with olive oil spray.

Using a food processor, or a plastic bag and a rolling pin, crush cereal into coarse crumbs. Add pecans and seasonings.

Remove chicken from marinade and shake off excess. Roll chicken in pecan mixture until coated on all sides. Place on the prepared baking sheet.

Bake for 25 minutes, until chicken is tender and juices are clear when pricked with a fork.

(continued)

Pecan-Crusted Chicken *(continued)*

PER SERVING: 274 calories; 8 g fat (26.4% calories from fat); 30 g protein; 18 g carbohydrate; 1 g dietary fiber; 67 mg cholesterol; 483 mg sodium. EXCHANGES: 1 grain (starch); 3½ lean meat; ½ non-fat milk; 1 fat.

Note

Pecans and other nuts contain heart-healthy omega-6 fatty acids. In one study, eating a handful of pecans daily for eight weeks resulted in a 16.5 percent drop in participants' average cholesterol levels.

Lemon-Mustard Chicken Breasts

*Marinate the night before, and this dish will be
on the table in 25 minutes.*

MAKES 4 SERVINGS   PREPARATION TIME: 2 HOURS 30 MINUTES

- 2 cloves garlic, peeled and minced
- ⅓ cup lemon juice
- ⅓ cup Dijon mustard
- 1 tablespoon extra-virgin olive oil
- ¼ teaspoon Low-Sodium Seasoned Salt (page 297) or salt substitute
- 4 (4-ounce) skinless, boneless chicken breast halves

Mix garlic, lemon juice, mustard, olive oil, and salt in a large, shallow bowl.

Place chicken in marinade, turn to coat both sides, and refrigerate, for at least 2 hours or overnight, turning chicken occasionally. (Or place chicken and marinade in a plastic bag, press out air, seal tightly, and marinate in the refrigerator. Turn bag occasionally to evenly coat chicken.)

Preheat a grill or broiler to high and place the grill or broiler pan 3 to 4 inches from heat.

Baste chicken with marinade and cook for 7 to 9 minutes. Turn, baste other side, and continue cooking for another 7 to 9 minutes, until done. (Juices will run clear when pricked with a fork.)

PER SERVING: 182 calories; 6 g fat (28.7% calories from fat); 28 g protein; 4 g carbohydrate; 1 g dietary fiber; 68 mg cholesterol; 413 mg sodium. EXCHANGES: 4 lean meat; 1 fat.

Note
When you're in a hurry, you can reduce the marinating time. The flavor may be a little less intense, but still tasty.

Mexican Casserole

*Lean ground turkey reduces the saturated
fat content of this easy casserole.*

MAKES 6 SERVINGS   PREPARATION TIME: 1 HOUR

Olive oil spray
1 pound ground lean turkey
2 cloves garlic, peeled and minced
1 medium onion, chopped
½ large green bell pepper, chopped
1 (14½-ounce) can Mexican-style stewed tomatoes
1 (15-ounce) can black or pinto beans, cooked, rinsed, and drained,
   or 1½ cups cooked dried beans
1 large can chopped green chiles (7 ounces), drained
2 tablespoons tomato paste
1 tablespoon chili powder
¾ cup grated Cheddar cheese
2 tablespoons freshly chopped cilantro

Heat a large nonstick skillet over medium heat. Spray with olive oil
spray and add turkey, garlic, onion, and green pepper. Cook, stirring occasionally and breaking up turkey with wooden spoon,
until turkey is browned, about 10 minutes.

Add tomatoes, beans, chiles, tomato paste, and chili powder to skillet. Reduce heat and simmer, stirring occasionally, for 8 to 10 minutes until most of the liquid has evaporated, but mixture is not dry.

Preheat the oven to 350 degrees F. Spray a medium-sized, covered
baking dish with olive oil spray.

Spoon mixture into the baking dish. Top with cheese and cover.

Bake for 20 minutes until hot and bubbly. Remove cover and bake another 5 minutes. Remove from the oven and sprinkle with cilantro.

PER SERVING: 220 calories; 11 g fat (42.5% calories from fat); 22 g protein; 11 g carbohydrate; 3 g dietary fiber; 64 mg cholesterol; 313 mg sodium. EXCHANGES: ½ grain (starch); 3 lean meat; 1½ vegetable; ½ fat.

SERVING IDEA: Serve this with Mary's Fresh Salsa (page 283) or Quick and Easy Salsa (page 284) and Tex-Mex Corn Salad (page 134).

Note
Replacing saturated fat with healthful mono- and polyunsaturated fats affects more than your risk of heart attack. A 2003 study found that people who ate the most saturated fat, found primarily in meat and dairy products, had more than double the risk of developing Alzheimer's disease as those eating little saturated fat.

Fish and Seafood

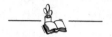

Canned tuna is the only fish many Americans ever eat. If you're one of them, you're not only missing out on a wealth of health benefits, but also on tasty culinary delights. Cold water fish such as salmon, mackerel, and sardines are our richest source of omega-3 fatty acids, which modulate inflammation and protect against heart disease, concerns for virtually all diabetics. Although other species contain fewer of these essential fats, all fish and seafood are low in saturated fat and abundant in protein, vitamins, and minerals. And once you try these fish recipes, you'll know what we mean by tasty culinary delights.

Many people are intimidated by cooking fish—it's great in a restaurant, but never seems to turn out as well at home. There is an art to cooking fish, and it's easy to master. First, purchase high-quality fish. Fresh is best (look for firm, almost translucent steaks and fillets), but frozen is also acceptable (keep bags of shelled, deveined, and cleaned raw shrimp and filleted fish in your freezer). Before cooking defrosted fish, dry it carefully with paper towels. Once fish is purchased or defrosted, use it within a day or two. Second, spice it up. Most types of fish are rather bland, so marinating them before cooking or topping with a sauce dramatically enhances flavor.

Third, don't overcook fish. The basic rule of thumb is ten minutes for each inch of fish, so a half-inch-thick fillet would only take five minutes. Average cooking times, depending on thickness, are as follows: outdoor grill (medium to medium-high heat), four to seven minutes per side; broiler (high heat), two to four minutes, turning only if fish is thick; stovetop (high heat), sauté one to three minutes per side; oven (medium to medium-high heat), bake fillets ten to fifteen minutes; George Foreman grill, three to seven minutes; poaching (simmering in water or stock), three to seven minutes. Whole fish take longer to cook.

The cooking times in the recipes in this chapter are guidelines. Fish is done when it turns from translucent to opaque and springs back lightly when you touch it (rather than leaving a fingerprint).

A final word on fish. Stay away from shark, swordfish, king mackerel, tilefish, and other large, predatory species, for they may contain high levels of mercury. Also, go easy on canned tuna—limit your intake to no more than one can a week. The fish and seafood we've recommended in this cookbook are safe.

Teriyaki Salmon

A favorite of salmon lovers.

MAKES 4 SERVINGS   PREPARATION TIME: 1 HOUR 20 MINUTES

¼ cup low-sodium soy sauce
¼ cup water
1 tablespoon rice vinegar
1 teaspoon xylitol or sugar
2 cloves garlic, peeled and minced
1 tablespoon gingerroot, peeled and minced, or 1 teaspoon ground
   ginger
1 pound salmon fillet, cut into 4-ounce fillets

Make marinade by combining soy sauce, water, vinegar, xylitol, garlic, and ginger in a small bowl, stirring until the xylitol dissolves.

Place salmon fillets and marinade in a plastic bag, remove air, seal, and place in the refrigerator for at least one hour or overnight, turning occasionally. (Or marinate in a covered dish.)

Preheat the broiler to high.

Remove salmon from marinade and place on an oiled rack, 2 or 3 inches from the heat source. Cook 2 to 4 minutes on each side (depending on thickness), turning once and brushing with the reserved marinade. (If fillets are very thin, do not turn.) Fish will be done when the flesh is opaque and springs back slightly to your touch. Do not overcook. You may also cook this on an outdoor grill, 4 to 7 minutes per side, or on a George Foreman grill, 4 to 7 minutes, depending on thickness of fish.

PER SERVING: 147 calories; 4 g fat (24.6% calories from fat); 24 g protein; 3 g carbohydrate; trace dietary fiber; 59 mg cholesterol; 340 mg sodium. EXCHANGES: 3 lean meat; ½ vegetable.

SERVING IDEA: Turn this into a light, yet satisfying main dish salad by serving each fillet atop a bed of salad greens.

Note
Make a point to eat salmon once or twice a week. The omega-3 fatty acids in this cold water fish reduce your risk of heart disease, fight inflammation, and improve mood and memory.

Spicy Salmon Cakes
The health benefits of salmon—from a can.

MAKES 4 SERVINGS (8 PATTIES)   PREPARATION TIME: 1 HOUR 20 MINUTES

1   large (14¾-ounce) can salmon, drained
⅓   cup finely chopped onion
⅓   cup finely chopped celery
¼   cup nonfat mayonnaise
1   teaspoon lemon juice
1   tablespoon Mrs. Dash salt-free seasoning
¼   teaspoon freshly ground black pepper
½   teaspoon Worcestershire sauce
    Dash Tabasco sauce
1   egg white, lightly beaten
⅓   cup bread crumbs (preferably sprouted-grain)
    Olive oil spray

Place salmon in a medium mixing bowl and carefully flake, discarding bones, skin, etc.

In another mixing bowl, combine onion, celery, mayonnaise, lemon juice, seasonings, egg white, and bread crumbs. Stir well. Gently fold into salmon, stirring carefully so salmon doesn't break up.

Measure a scant ¼ cup salmon mixture and form into a flat patty. Repeat with remaining salmon. Refrigerate, covered, for 1 hour.

Heat a large nonstick skillet over medium heat. Spray with olive oil spray and place salmon cakes in the hot skillet. Flatten slightly with spatula. Cook for about 4 minutes, turn, and cook 4 minutes on the other side, or until golden brown. Gently remove from the skillet with a spatula and place on serving plates. (They will be a bit fragile.)

PER SERVING: 181 calories; 4 g fat (21.2% calories from fat); 23 g protein; 11 g carbohydrate; 1 g dietary fiber; 54 mg cholesterol; 367 mg sodium. EXCHANGES: ½ grain (starch); 3 lean meat; ½ vegetable.

SERVING IDEA: One way to serve Spicy Salmon Cakes is as a main dish salad. Pile individual serving plates high with cleaned spinach leaves or mixed lettuce and top with two salmon patties. Top with Tangy Tartar Sauce (page 285) thinned with a little milk. Delicious!

Note
Make a double batch and serve leftovers as a snack or sandwich filling.

Baked Salmon Dijon

An easy way to prepare fish.

MAKES 4 SERVINGS   PREPARATION TIME: 25 MINUTES

   Olive oil spray
 2 *teaspoons extra-virgin olive oil*
1½ *tablespoons Dijon mustard*
 2 *tablespoons lemon juice*
1½ *tablespoons chopped chives (fresh or freeze-dried) or parsley*
 1 *teaspoon grated lemon peel*
 ¼ *teaspoon salt or salt substitute*
 ⅛ *teaspoon freshly ground black pepper*
 1 *pound salmon fillet, cut into 4-ounce fillets*

Preheat the oven to 400 degrees F. Spray a large baking dish with olive oil spray.

Combine olive oil, mustard, lemon juice, chives, lemon peel, salt, and pepper and stir until well blended.

Rub oil-mustard mixture over both sides of salmon. Place in baking dish (skin side down if not skinned). Bake for 12 to 15 minutes, depending on thickness.

Transfer to serving plates and spoon pan juices over fillets.

PER SERVING: 159 calories; 6 g fat (37.4% calories from fat); 23 g protein; 1 g carbohydrate; trace dietary fiber; 59 mg cholesterol; 280 mg sodium. EXCHANGES: 3 lean meat; ½ fat.

Note

If you have the choice, pick fresh, wild salmon from Alaska or the Pacific Northwest over farm-raised Atlantic salmon. It hasn't been exposed to antibiotics or pesticides, and it comes by its pink color and health-enhancing omega-3 fatty acids naturally.

Gourmet Fish Sticks

Nothing like the frozen fish sticks from your childhood.

MAKES 4 SERVINGS   PREPARATION TIME: 40 MINUTES

1   cup Kellogg's Special K cereal or dry bread crumbs
4   tablespoons low-fat mayonnaise
1   tablespoon lemon juice
1   pound halibut or grouper or other firm fish fillet
¼   teaspoon seasoned salt
¼   teaspoon freshly ground black pepper
    Olive oil spray

Crush cereal by placing in a plastic bag and rolling a can or rolling pin over the bag. Repeat until finely crushed. You may also use a blender or food processor.

Preheat the oven to 425 degrees F.

Mix mayonnaise, lemon juice, salt, and pepper in a small bowl.

Cut fish into ¾- to 1-inch-wide strips. Dip each strip in mayonnaise mixture, then dredge in cereal or bread crumbs. Place on a baking sheet sprayed with olive oil spray. Bake for 10 to 15 minutes, until fish is firm and coating is lightly browned.

PER SERVING: 194 calories; 7 g fat (32.9% calories from fat); 24 g protein; 7 g carbohydrate; trace dietary fiber; 41 mg cholesterol; 272 mg sodium. EXCHANGES: ½ grain (starch); 3½ lean meat; 1 fat.

SERVING IDEA: Serve this with Tangy Tartar Sauce (page 285).

Broiled Fish Fillets
with Cucumber-Dill Sauce

From fridge to table in 15 minutes.

MAKES 4 SERVINGS   PREPARATION TIME: 15 MINUTES

1 *pound cod or pollock or other thin fillets, cut into 4-ounce fillets*
2 *teaspoons extra-virgin olive oil*
¼ *teaspoon Low-Sodium Seasoned Salt (page 297) or salt substitute*
   Dash freshly ground black pepper
1 *cup Cucumber-Dill Sauce (page 278)*

Preheat the broiler and arrange an oven rack 5 or 6 inches from the heating element.

Dry fish and rub both sides with olive oil. Sprinkle with salt and pepper.

Cook 2 to 3 minutes, depending on thickness. (Turning is not necessary unless fish is thick.) When the fish is opaque and lightly springs back when you touch it, it is done. Be careful not to overcook.

Serve with Cucumber-Dill Sauce.

PER SERVING (includes Cucumber-Dill Sauce): 135 calories; 3 g fat (28.3% calories from fat); 22 g protein; 3 g carbohydrate; trace dietary fiber; 50 mg cholesterol; 265 mg sodium. EXCHANGES: 2½ lean meat; ½ fat.

Note
Broiling is an easy way to prepare any kind of fish. The only trick is to not overcook. Thin fillets may require only 2 to 3 minutes total. If you are broiling thicker fillets or steaks, turn them after 3 to 5 minutes and continue cooking.

Blackened Cajun Catfish

Straight from New Orleans.

MAKES 4 SERVINGS   PREPARATION TIME: 15 MINUTES

2   *teaspoons paprika*
1   *teaspoon ground cumin*
1   *teaspoon chili powder*
1   *teaspoon onion powder*
1   *teaspoon dried oregano*
1   *teaspoon dried garlic powder*
1   *teaspoon dried thyme*
½   *teaspoon salt or salt substitute*
¼   *teaspoon freshly ground black pepper*
¼   *teaspoon cayenne pepper, or to taste*
1   *pound skinned catfish or other fish cut into 4-ounce fillets*
1   *tablespoon extra-virgin olive oil*
4   *parsley sprigs, for garnish*
4   *lemon wedges*

Combine spices, mix well, and spread on a plate.

Preheat a heavy skillet (preferably cast-iron, or stainless-steel) over medium heat until just short of smoking, about 5 minutes. (See Note.)

Brush both sides of fish fillets with olive oil, then dip into spices, coating well on both sides.

Cook quickly in the hot skillet until blackened. Flip over and cook other side. This will take only 1 to 2 minutes per side for thin fillets, a little longer for thicker ones. Sprinkle with parsley sprigs and serve with lemon wedges.

(continued)

Blackened Cajun Catfish (continued)

PER SERVING: 154 calories; 7 g fat (41.0% calories from fat); 19 g protein; 4 g carbohydrate; 1 g dietary fiber; 66 mg cholesterol; 324 mg sodium. EXCHANGES: 2½ lean meat; 1 fat.

SERVING IDEA: Serve this on a bed of salad greens, topped with Garlic Vinaigrette salad dressing (page 274).

Note
If you use the traditional method of blackening, make sure your stove fan is on (this gets smoky) and your scouring pad ready for cleaning the pan. Blackened catfish may also be grilled or broiled. Cooking time will vary from 4 to 7 minutes per side for grilling and 2 to 4 minutes for broiling.

Baked Trout with Mushrooms and Onions

A clean and easy method of preparing whole fish.

MAKES 4 SERVINGS   PREPARATION TIME: 50 MINUTES

Olive oil spray

4 ½-pound or 2 1-pound whole (head and tail intact) rainbow trout, cleaned

2 tablespoons lemon juice

2 tablespoons freshly chopped parsley

1 tablespoon extra-virgin olive oil

1 onion, thinly sliced

1 clove garlic, peeled and minced

2 cups thinly sliced fresh mushrooms

½ teaspoon salt or salt substitute

¼ teaspoon freshly ground black pepper

Preheat the oven to 350 degrees F.

Spray the bottom of a large, shallow ovenproof dish with olive oil spray and place trout side by side in the dish. Sprinkle lemon juice and 1 tablespoon parsley on fish, cover with foil, and bake 20 to 30 minutes, until the fish are tender and flaky.

Meanwhile, heat olive oil in a nonstick skillet over medium heat. Add onions and garlic and cook for 5 minutes, stirring occasionally. Add mushrooms, salt, and pepper, and cook, stirring, another 3 to 5 minutes. Remove from heat. Reheat just before serving.

Place trout on serving plates and top each with mushroom-onion mixture and remaining parsley.

(continued)

Baked Trout with Mushrooms and Onions (continued)

PER SERVING: 289 calories; 10 g fat (32.9% calories from fat); 42 g protein; 5 g carbohydrate; 1 g dietary fiber; 113 mg cholesterol; 324 mg sodium. EXCHANGES: 6 lean meat; 1 vegetable; ½ fat.

Note
Baked whole fish makes a beautiful presentation but is a challenge to eat. To remove the bones before serving, cut along the backbone from the neck to the tail. Loosen the top fillet from the bone and flip it over to the side. Lift the bone out from the tail and remove any small bones that remain. If fish breaks during this process, put it back together and cover with sauce.

Honey Glazed Mahimahi

Glazed with a touch of sweetness.

MAKES 4 SERVINGS   PREPARATION TIME: 50 MINUTES

3 tablespoons brown rice syrup or honey
3 tablespoons rice vinegar
2 tablespoons low-sodium soy sauce
1 teaspoon gingerroot, peeled and grated, or ½ teaspoon ground
   ginger
2 cloves garlic, peeled and minced
1 pound mahimahi (dolphin fish) or ahi tuna, cut into 4-ounce
   fillets
1½ teaspoons extra-virgin olive oil

Mix brown rice syrup, rice vinegar, soy sauce, ginger, and garlic in a small bowl.

Wash and dry fish, place in a covered bowl, and pour marinade over fish, turning fillets to coat evenly. (Or place marinade and fillets in a plastic bag, squeeze out the air, and seal.) Marinate in the refrigerator for at least 30 minutes, turning fish or the bag occasionally.

Heat olive oil over medium-high heat in a nonstick skillet. Remove fish from marinade and cook in skillet, 2 to 3 minutes. Turn and cook an additional 2 to 3 minutes. Remove and keep warm.

Add remaining marinade to the skillet and cook over medium-high heat for about 1 minute, stirring constantly with a wooden spoon. Pour over fish and serve.

PER SERVING: 182 calories; 2 g fat (11.9% calories from fat); 22 g protein; 19 g carbohydrate; trace dietary fiber; 83 mg cholesterol; 417 mg sodium. EXCHANGES: 3 lean meat; ½ vegetable; ½ fat.

Halibut with Artichoke Salsa

Fast and full of flavor.

MAKES 4 SERVINGS   PREPARATION TIME: 15 MINUTES

Olive oil spray
1 *pound halibut, cut into 4 4-ounce fillets*
2 *teaspoons extra-virgin olive oil*
¼ *teaspoon salt or salt substitute*
¼ *teaspoon freshly ground black pepper*
1 *cup Artichoke Salsa (page 282)*

Preheat the broiler or grill. Spray the broiler pan or grill with olive oil spray.

Brush both sides of halibut with olive oil and season with salt and pepper.

Place on the broiler pan or grill and cook, 2 to 3 inches from heat source, for 2 to 4 minutes, until fish is opaque and top is lightly browned. If steaks are very thick, turn after 3 minutes and cook 2 to 3 minutes on other side.

PER SERVING (includes Artichoke Salsa): 190 calories; 7 g fat (75.5% calories from fat); 26 g protein; 5 g carbohydrate; 2 g dietary fiber; 36 mg cholesterol; 352 mg sodium. EXCHANGES: 3½ lean meat; 1 fat.

Note
Line the broiler pan with aluminum foil for easier cleanup.

Marinated Fish Fillets in Parchment Paper

Eating fish in parchment is like opening a gift at the table.

MAKES 4 SERVINGS   PREPARATION TIME: 1 HOUR

1 tablespoon extra-virgin olive oil
2 tablespoons lime juice
1 teaspoon grated lime peel
2 teaspoons Dijon mustard
1 tablespoon freshly chopped parsley
1 tablespoon freshly chopped cilantro
½ teaspoon salt or salt substitute
¼ teaspoon freshly ground black pepper
1 pound cod fillet, cut into 4-ounce boneless, skinless pieces
 Parchment paper or waxed paper (in a pinch)

Combine olive oil, lime juice, lime peel, mustard, parsley, cilantro, salt, and pepper in a small bowl and mix well.

Place fish in a shallow dish and pour marinade over fillets, turning to coat. Cover, and place in the refrigerator to marinate for 30 minutes, turning occasionally. (You may also place fish and marinade in a plastic bag, squeeze out the air, and seal. Turn the bag occasionally.)

Preheat the oven to 400 degrees F. Prepare 4 sheets parchment paper (or a double-thickness waxed paper). Each should be large enough to wrap around 1 piece of fish.

Place 1 piece of fish in the middle of each piece of parchment paper and spoon one-fourth of remaining marinade over fish. Bring the ends of the paper together to cover fish, then fold the edges together to tightly secure the packet. Repeat with the remaining fillets.

(continued)

Marinated Fish Fillets in Parchment Paper *(continued)*

Place on a baking sheet and cook for 10 to 15 minutes, until fish is tender. Serve in paper so diners can open these delightfully aromatic packets at the table.

PER SERVING: 132 calories; 4 g fat (29.7% calories from fat); 21 g protein; 2 g carbohydrate; trace dietary fiber; 49 mg cholesterol; 361 mg sodium. EXCHANGES: 2½ lean meat; ½ fat.

SERVING IDEA: Marinated Fish Fillets go well with Moroccan Couscous (page 271) and Garlicky Spinach (page 254).

Notes
Poisson en papillote ("fish in parchment paper") is a classic French dish with many variations. Try it with other types of fish topped with your choice of herbs and vegetables.

Grilled Shrimp Brochettes

Shrimp on a skewer in a delightful marinade.

MAKES 4 SERVINGS   PREPARATION TIME: 50 MINUTES

 3 *tablespoons lime juice*
 1 *tablespoon extra-virgin olive oil*
 1 *tablespoon low-sodium soy sauce or salt substitute*
 ¼ *teaspoon freshly ground black pepper*
 ¼ *teaspoon paprika*
 ⅛ *teaspoon red pepper flakes*
 1 *pound (20 to 25) large shrimp, peeled, deveined, and rinsed, tails on (see Note)*
 4 *(10- to 12-inch) bamboo skewers*
    Olive oil spray
 4 *lime wedges*

Combine lime juice, olive oil, soy sauce, black pepper, paprika, and red pepper flakes and mix well.

Place cleaned shrimp and marinade in a covered bowl, stir well to coat all shrimp, and refrigerate for at least 30 minutes, stirring occasionally. (Or place marinade and shrimp in a plastic bag, squeeze out the air, seal, and refrigerate.)

Soak bamboo skewers in water for at least 30 minutes.

Preheat the grill or broiler. Spray the grill or broiler tray with olive oil spray.

(continued)

Grilled Shrimp Brochettes (continued)

Remove shrimp from marinade and thread onto bamboo skewers, leaving a little space between each shrimp. Baste with marinade. Grill 2 to 3 minutes or broil 1 to 2 minutes until pink, turn, and cook another 2 to 3 minutes.

Serve with lime wedges.

PER SERVING: 161 calories; 5 g fat (30.3% calories from fat); 23 g protein; 4 g carbohydrate; trace dietary fiber; 173 mg cholesterol; 319 mg sodium. EXCHANGES: 3 lean meat; ½ fat.

SERVING IDEA: This goes well with Thai Noodles (page 272) and a green salad.

Note

In recipes calling for shrimp, you can use fresh or frozen raw shrimp. We suggest keeping bags of frozen, uncooked shrimp in your freezer. If they are already peeled and deveined, so much the better. If not, defrost the shrimp if needed, then using your fingers, start at the large end and peel off the shells. Leave the tails intact, if you want. To devein, take a paring knife and make a shallow cut down the length of the back of each shrimp. Wash out the exposed vein under running water.

Shrimp Creole

Colorful, fragrant, and yummy.

MAKES 4 SERVINGS   PREPARATION TIME: 25 MINUTES

1   *teaspoon extra-virgin olive oil*
½   *large green bell pepper, cut into 1-inch pieces*
1   *onion, cut into 1-inch pieces*
2   *cloves garlic, peeled and minced*
¾   *pound (20 to 35) large or medium shrimp, peeled, deveined, and rinsed, tails removed*
1   *(14½-ounce) can low-sodium tomatoes with juice, chopped*
1   *teaspoon freshly chopped thyme or ¼ teaspoon dried thyme*
½   *teaspoon freshly ground black pepper*
¼   *teaspoon Low-Sodium Seasoned Salt (page 297) or salt substitute*
⅛   *teaspoon red pepper flakes*

Heat olive oil in a large nonstick skillet over medium-high heat. Add green pepper, onion, and garlic and cook for 3 minutes, stirring occasionally, until crisp-tender.

Stir in shrimp, tomatoes, thyme, black pepper, salt, and red pepper flakes. Bring to a boil, then reduce heat. Cover and simmer 4 to 6 minutes, stirring occasionally, until shrimp are pink and firm.

PER SERVING: 138 calories; 3 g fat (18.2% calories from fat); 19 g protein; 9 g carbohydrate; 2 g dietary fiber; 129 mg cholesterol; 223 mg sodium. EXCHANGES: 2½ lean meat; 1½ vegetable.

SERVING IDEA: Serve this over barley, quinoa, or long-grain brown rice (½ cup per serving).

Scampi in Wine and Garlic Sauce

As good as in any restaurant.

MAKES 4 SERVINGS   PREPARATION TIME: 25 MINUTES

3 large cloves garlic, peeled and minced
1 tablespoon extra-virgin olive oil
1 pound (20 to 25) large shrimp peeled, deveined, and rinsed, tails removed
½ cup dry white wine or extra-dry vermouth
3 teaspoons lemon juice
1 tablespoon freshly chopped parsley
Pinch dried oregano
¼ teaspoon salt or salt substitute
¼ teaspoon freshly ground black pepper
Parsley sprigs, for garnish

In a large skillet over medium heat, lightly sauté garlic in olive oil for 1 minute. Add shrimp to the skillet and continue cooking, stirring and turning, until shrimp just turns pink, 2 to 3 minutes. Remove from the skillet.

Turn up the heat to high and add wine, lemon juice, parsley, oregano, salt, and pepper. Bring to a boil and cook for 3 to 4 minutes, until sauce is reduced by half.

Reduce the heat to medium, return shrimp to the skillet and cook, stirring for 1 to 2 minutes, until shrimp is heated through.

Remove to serving plates and sprinkle with parsley.

PER SERVING: 175 calories; 5 g fat (31.9% calories from fat); 23 g protein; 2 g carbohydrate; trace dietary fiber; 173 mg cholesterol; 304 mg sodium. EXCHANGES: 3 lean meat; ½ fat.

Note

Extra-dry vermouth is always a good choice in recipes calling for white wine.

Stir-Fried Scallops and Snow Peas

A meal unto itself.

MAKES 4 SERVINGS   PREPARATION TIME: 25 MINUTES

 4 *ounces vermicelli or other thin pasta, broken into 3- to-4-inch pieces*
 ½ *cup water*
 2 *tablespoons low-sodium soy sauce*
 2 *tablespoons dry sherry or apple juice*
 1 *teaspoon cornstarch*
 1 *teaspoon grated gingerroot or ½ teaspoon ground ginger*
 ⅛ *teaspoon red pepper flakes*
 ¾ *pound sea scallops or bay scallops*
 2 *teaspoons extra-virgin olive oil*
 3 *cloves garlic, peeled and minced*
 3 *cups snow peas*
 1 *red bell pepper, cut into ¼-by-1-inch strips*
 2 *green onions, shredded*

Cook vermicelli in 4 cups of rapidly boiling water until just tender (al dente), about 5 minutes. Do not overcook. Drain, rinse, and set aside.

Meanwhile, combine water, soy sauce, sherry, cornstarch, ginger, and pepper flakes in a small bowl.

If you're using large sea scallops, cut into quarters.

Heat 1 teaspoon olive oil in a wok or large skillet over medium heat. Add garlic and stir-fry, stirring constantly, for 15 seconds. Add snow peas and red pepper and stir-fry for 5 minutes. Remove from the wok.

Add remaining teaspoon of olive oil to the wok, then add scallops and stir-fry for 2 to 3 minutes until opaque. Return peas and red peppers to the wok and cook, stirring for 1 to 2 minutes. Add vermicelli and stir.

Stir sauce and pour into the wok. Cook, stirring constantly, until sauce is thick and vermicelli is heated through, about 3 minutes.

Top with shredded green onions.

PER SERVING: 245 calories; 3 g fat (12.0% calories from fat); 19 g protein; 32 g carbohydrate; 2 g dietary fiber; 28 mg cholesterol; 443 mg sodium. EXCHANGES: 1½ grain (starch); 2 lean meat; 1½ vegetable; ½ fat.

SERVING IDEA: This goes well with Mandarin Salad (page 131).

Linguine with Clam Sauce

Canned clams make this quick and easy.

MAKES 4 SERVINGS   PREPARATION TIME: 25 MINUTES

5 ounces linguine
2 (6½-ounce) cans clams with juice
½ tablespoon extra-virgin olive oil
3 cloves garlic, peeled and minced
⅛ teaspoon crushed red pepper flakes
¼ cup freshly chopped parsley
¼ cup grated Parmesan cheese

Cook linguine in boiling water per package instructions until al dente, or just tender, about 8 to 10 minutes. Drain, place in a large serving bowl, and keep warm.

Meanwhile, strain juice from clams into a small saucepan. Simmer clam juice over medium-high heat until liquid is reduced by half.

In a small skillet, heat olive oil over medium heat. Add garlic and cook, stirring continuously, for 1 minute, until garlic is translucent. Add pepper flakes and the reduced clam juice, bring to a boil, and add clams. Cook for another minute until heated through.

Pour sauce over hot linguine and toss, along with parsley. Top with Parmesan cheese.

PER SERVING: 261 calories; 5 g fat (17% calories from fat); 20 g protein; 33 g carbohydrate; 1 g dietary fiber; 37 mg cholesterol; 267 mg sodium. EXCHANGES: 2 grain (starch); lean meat; ½ fat; ½ other carbohydrates.

Note
Pasta cooked al dente (barely done) has a lower glycemic index and a less dramatic effect on blood sugar.

Vegetarian

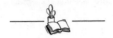

A vegetarian diet, with its emphasis on fiber-rich whole grains, vegetables, and other plant foods, is associated with a reduced risk of developing diabetes. But does such a diet have a role in the treatment of existing diabetes? Absolutely! A varied vegetarian diet can provide high-quality protein, healthy fats, and fiber-rich, low-glycemic carbohydrates that allow for good glucose control.

The meatless main dishes in this section are balanced in terms of calories and proportions of fat, protein, and carbohydrates—but over the top in taste and ease of preparation. A few dishes include tofu (Curried Vegetables with Tofu, page 237, and Mushroom Madness, page 235), but most are made with more familiar pasta (Lasagna Roll-Ups, page 223, and Angel Hair Pasta with Fresh Basil, Tomatoes, and Garlic, page 222) and vegetables (Stuffed Peppers Provençale, page 245, and Zen Stir-Fry, page 239).

Even if you're not a vegetarian, we hope you'll try these recipes. If you are vegetarian, please note that many of the recipes in other chapters of this book are meatless, and those that are not may be modified. (For example, replace chicken breasts with tofu or soy "chicken" cutlets and patties available in health food stores.)

Angel Hair Pasta with
Fresh Basil, Tomatoes, and Garlic

A favorite recipe for summer, when tomatoes and basil are at their prime.

MAKES 4 SERVINGS   PREPARATION TIME: 1 HOUR 15 MINUTES

1½ cups chopped fresh tomatoes (preferably Roma)
 1 cup freshly chopped basil
½ cup freshly chopped parsley
 3 cloves garlic, peeled and minced
 2 tablespoons extra-virgin olive oil
¼ teaspoon salt or salt substitute
¼ teaspoon red pepper flakes
 6 ounces angel hair pasta (capellini) or other thin pasta
⅓ cup grated Parmesan cheese

Place tomatoes, basil, and parsley in a medium glass mixing bowl and stir in garlic, olive oil, salt, and pepper flakes. Mix well and marinate at room temperature for an hour. (If you plan to serve it later, refrigerate and bring to room temperature before serving.)

Cook pasta in boiling water per package directions or al dente (until barely done and firm to the bite), about 4 minutes. Drain.

Transfer hot pasta to a large serving dish. Toss with tomato mixture and Parmesan cheese. Serve at once.

PER SERVING: 271 calories; 10 g fat (32% calories from fat); 9 g protein; 37 g carbohydrate; 2 g dietary fiber; 5 mg cholesterol; 271 mg sodium. EXCHANGES: 2 grain (starch); ½ lean meat; 1 vegetable; 1½ fat.

Note
If you like pasta, but it raises your blood sugar, try the low-carb, high-protein varieties sold in health food stores.

Lasagna Roll-Ups

A new look for an old favorite.

MAKES 4 SERVINGS   PREPARATION TIME: 1 HOUR 20 MINUTES

4 ounces (6 noodles) lasagna
1 teaspoon extra-virgin olive oil
1 cup coarsely chopped broccoli florets
1 cup thinly sliced mushrooms
1 cup chopped onion
8 ounces nonfat ricotta cheese
2 ounces (½ cup) part skim milk mozzarella cheese grated
¼ cup freshly chopped parsley
   Olive oil spray
2 cups Homemade Marinara Sauce (page 294) or bottled spaghetti
   sauce or Tomato Cream Sauce (page 290)

Cook lasagna per package directions, boiling just until barely tender, about 10 minutes. Drain, rinse, separate, and cut each noodle in half. Set aside.

Prepare filling by heating olive oil in a medium skillet over medium heat. Add broccoli, mushrooms, and onion and cook, stirring frequently, for 5 or 6 minutes, until broccoli is tender. Transfer to a medium mixing bowl, cool briefly, then add cheeses and parsley, stirring well.

Preheat the oven to 350 degrees F. Spray an 8-by-8-inch baking dish with olive oil spray.

Spoon ½ cup of the marinara sauce into the bottom of the prepared baking dish. Spread ⅓ cup of filling over length of a lasagna noodle, then roll up, beginning with one of the short ends. Place, seam side

(continued)

Lasagna Roll-Ups *(continued)*

down,in the baking dish. Repeat with remaining lasagna. Spoon re-maining 1½ cups of sauce over lasagna roll-ups.

Cover and bake for 40 minutes. Remove cover and bake 10 more minutes, until roll-ups are heated all the way through.

PER SERVING: 255 calories; 4 g fat (14.6% calories from fat); 18 g protein; 37 g carbohydrate; 4 g dietary fiber; 17 mg cholesterol; 381 mg sodium. EXCHANGES: 1½ grain (starch); 1½ lean meat; 2½ vegetable; ½ fat.

Note

Broccoli is a nutritional powerhouse, containing an array of phy-tonutrients that boost your detox system and protect against cancer. If you're not a broccoli fan, substitute 3 cups fresh spinach (cleaned, stems removed, coarsely chopped) or a 10-ounce package of frozen spinach (defrosted and with moisture squeezed out) and add to the skillet during the last 3 minutes of cooking the filling.

Eggplant-Zucchini Parmesan

A healthier version of an Italian classic.

MAKES 6 SERVINGS   PREPARATION TIME: 1 HOUR 10 MINUTES

1 *pound (3 medium) zucchini*
1 *medium eggplant*
  Olive oil spray
2½ *cups Homemade Marinara Sauce (page 294) or bottled spaghetti*
  sauce
4 *ounces part skim milk mozzarella cheese, grated*
½ *cup freshly grated Parmesan cheese*
6 *ounces rigatoni or pasta of your choice*
1 *teaspoon extra-virgin olive oil*
2 *tablespoons freshly chopped parsley*

Slice zucchini into ½-inch slices. Peel eggplant and cut into ½-inch slices, then into 1-inch pieces.

Heat a large nonstick skillet over medium heat. Spray with olive oil spray, then add eggplant and zucchini in batches. Turn after 3 minutes, or when lightly browned, and brown the other side for about 3 minutes. Repeat until all vegetables are browned.

Preheat the oven to 375 degrees F. Spray an 8-by-8-inch baking dish with olive oil spray.

Pour ½ cup of marinara sauce evenly into the baking dish. Spread eggplant evenly over sauce. Sprinkle one-third of each cheese over eggplant. Pour 1 cup of sauce evenly over eggplant and cheese. Layer zucchini evenly on sauce. Sprinkle with one-third of cheeses. Pour remaining 1 cup sauce over zucchini and top with remaining one-third of cheeses. Cover tightly.

(continued)

Eggplant-Zucchini Parmesan (continued)

Bake for 45 minutes, removing cover during last 10 minutes, until hot and bubbly.

While eggplant-zucchini dish is cooking, cook rigatoni in boiling water per package directions, about 10 minutes, just until tender (al dente). Drain, return to cooking pan, and toss with olive oil and parsley.

Serve side by side or top pasta with the eggplant-zucchini.

PER SERVING: 253 calories; 7 g fat (23.3% calories from fat); 14 g protein; 35 g carbohydrate; 5 g dietary fiber; 15 mg cholesterol; 386 mg sodium. EXCHANGES: 1½ grain (starch); 1 lean meat; 2½ vegetable; ½ fat.

SERVING IDEA: All you need is a salad to make this a complete meal.

Note
Many recipes call for salting eggplant and letting it sit 30 minutes before cooking to remove bitterness and to draw out moisture, making it less absorbent so it won't soak up so much oil when frying. Since eggplant really isn't bitter and none of our recipes uses a lot of oil for frying—plus we're cutting back on sodium—skip the salting.

Baked Chile Rellenos

If you love chile rellenos, you—and your waistline—
will like this lower-calorie version.

MAKES 4 SERVINGS   PREPARATION TIME: 1 HOUR

Olive oil spray
2   egg whites
1   egg
3   tablespoons nonfat milk
2   tablespoons unbleached flour
¼   teaspoon salt or salt substitute
Dash freshly ground black pepper
4   ounces Cheddar cheese
1½ (7-ounce) cans whole green chiles (8 chiles), drained

Preheat oven to 375 degrees F. Spray an 8-by-8-inch baking dish with olive oil spray.

Mix egg whites, egg, and milk in a small bowl and beat with an electric mixer or whisk for 30 to 60 seconds. Add flour, salt, and pepper, and continue beating for another minute.

Cut cheese into ½-inch-by-2-inch strips and stuff into chiles.

Place chiles in baking dish and pour egg mixture over top. Bake for 45 minutes, until eggs are puffy and cheese has melted.

PER SERVING: 162 calories; 11 g fat (58.4% calories from fat); 11 g protein; 6 g carbohydrate; trace dietary fiber; 77 mg cholesterol; 358 mg sodium. EXCHANGES: 1½ lean meat; ½ vegetable; 1½ fat.

SERVING IDEAS: Top with salsa, and serve with Texas Caviar (page 133) or Tex-Mex Corn Salad (page 134).

Cauliflower Croquettes
An unusual alternative to fish croquettes.

MAKES 4 SERVINGS   PREPARATION TIME: 1 HOUR

4 cups fresh cauliflower florets or 1 (16-ounce) package frozen
  cauliflower
2 tablespoons extra-virgin olive oil
3 tablespoons unbleached flour
¾ cup skim milk
1 egg
⅓ cup grated Parmesan cheese
2 tablespoons chopped fresh or freeze-dried chives
½ teaspoon garlic powder
½ teaspoon onion powder
1 egg white or ¼ Egg Beaters or other egg white product
⅓ cup bread crumbs (preferably sprouted-grain)
  Olive oil spray

Steam cauliflower over boiling water for 5 or 6 minutes or cook covered in a microwave with 2 to 3 tablespoons of water until tender. Drain and cool enough to handle, then chop finely.

Heat olive oil in a medium saucepan over medium heat, add flour and cook, stirring constantly, for 1 minute. Add milk and cook, stirring until very thick.

Turn off heat, stir in egg, cheese, chives, and seasonings. Mix well, then fold in cauliflower. Chill until cool, 15 minutes in the freezer or 30 minutes in the fridge.

Form cauliflower into 8 2½-inch patties. Dip into egg whites, then into bread crumbs.

Heat a large nonstick skillet over medium heat. Spray with olive oil. Cook croquettes in batches over medium heat 3 to 4 minutes on each side, turning carefully. Gently transfer to a serving plate.

PER SERVING: 208 calories; 11 g fat (44.9% calories from fat); 10 g protein; 19 g carbohydrate; 3 g dietary fiber; 53 mg cholesterol; 283 mg sodium. EXCHANGES: ½ grain (starch); ½ lean meat; 1 vegetable; 1½ fat.

SERVING IDEA: Serve with a hearty, protein-rich side dish such as Quinoa Pilaf (page 268) or Garbanzo Curry (page 266).

Note
Cauliflower, like broccoli, is a member of the cruciferous family of vegetables, which has been demonstrated to protect against cancer.

Broccoli-Cheddar Pie

Reduce fat and calories with a bread crumb crust.

MAKES 6 SERVINGS   PREPARATION TIME: 1 HOUR

2 cups fresh broccoli florets or 8 ounces frozen broccoli
   Olive oil spray
⅔ cup bread crumbs (preferably sprouted-grain, 1 slice crumbled
   in a food processor or blender)
1 tablespoon grated Parmesan cheese
1½ cups low-fat cottage cheese (preferably large curd)
¼ cup skim milk
1 cup grated low-sodium Cheddar cheese
6 egg whites or ¾ cup Egg Beaters or other egg white product
½ teaspoon dried tarragon
¼ teaspoon freshly ground black pepper

Steam broccoli for 5 minutes until tender-crisp, or cook in the
microwave for 3 minutes. Cool and coarsely chop. Set aside.

Meanwhile, preheat the oven to 350 degrees F. Spray a 9-inch pie
pan with olive oil spray.

Mix bread crumbs and Parmesan cheese in a small bowl. Press onto
the sides and bottom of the prepared pie pan.

Mix cottage cheese, milk, Cheddar cheese, egg whites, tarragon,
and pepper together. Stir in broccoli and pour into the pie pan.

Bake 55 to 65 minutes, or until set. (A knife inserted into pie
should come out clean.)

PER SERVING: 195 calories; 8 g fat (35.9% calories from fat); 18 g protein; 13 g carbohydrate; 1 g dietary fiber; 22 mg cholesterol; 419 mg
sodium. EXCHANGES: ½ grain (starch); 2 lean meat; 1 fat.

Vegetable-Tofu Shish Kebabs

A light, healthy change from the usual barbecue fare.

MAKES 4 SERVINGS   PREPARATION TIME: 1 HOUR

 3 *tablespoons low-sodium soy sauce*
 3 *tablespoons lemon juice*
 1 *tablespoon extra-virgin olive oil*
 1 *tablespoon rice wine or sherry*
 1 *tablespoon xylitol*
 ½ *teaspoon ground ginger*
 1 *clove garlic, peeled and minced*
14 *ounces (1 package) extra-firm tofu*
 1 *large onion, cut into 1-inch pieces*
16 *whole cherry tomatoes*
 1 *large green pepper, cut into 1-inch pieces*
 8 *fresh mushrooms*
    Olive oil spray

Soak 8 10- to 12-inch wooden skewers in water for 30 minutes.

Combine soy sauce, lemon juice, olive oil, rice wine, xylitol, ground ginger, and garlic and stir well. Divide into two bowls.

Drain tofu and dry with paper towels. Cut into ¾ to 1 inch cubes and place in one bowl of marinade. Place onion, tomatoes, pepper, and mushrooms in the other bowl. Cover both bowls and refrigerate for a minimum of 30 minutes; 1 or 2 hours is even better. Gently stir occasionally.

Heat grill to medium high.

(continued)

Vegetable-Tofu Shish Kebabs *(continued)*

Thread tofu alternating with vegetables on skewers and spray with olive oil. Reserve remaining marinade for basting.

Cook for 7 to 10 minutes, turning every 3 minutes or so and basting with reserved marinade.

PER SERVING: 172 calories; 8 g fat (39.5% calories from fat); 11 g protein; 18 g carbohydrate; 3 g dietary fiber; 0 mg cholesterol; 467 mg sodium. EXCHANGES: 2 lean meat; 2 vegetable; 1 fat.

Note
Make tofu a regular part of your diet. Like other soy products, it contains high-quality protein and little fat. It also lowers cholesterol, protects against free radical damage, and has potent anti-cancer activity. For dishes like this, use firm or extra-firm tofu.

Moussaka

A vegetarian version of a Greek standard.

MAKES 8 SERVINGS   PREPARATION TIME: 1 HOUR 45 MINUTES

1¼ cups dried lentils
  5 cups low-sodium vegetable stock or chicken stock
  1 bay leaf
  1 teaspoon extra-virgin olive oil
  1 medium onion, thinly sliced
  1 clove garlic, peeled and minced
  8 ounces mushrooms, sliced
  1 (14½-ounce) can low-sodium tomatoes, chopped, with juice
  2 tablespoons tomato paste
  ½ teaspoon dried oregano
  ½ teaspoon dried basil
  ¼ teaspoon ground cinnamon
  1 pound (1 large) eggplant, unpeeled
     Olive oil spray
1¼ cups nonfat plain yogurt
  4 egg whites or ½ cup Egg Beaters or other egg white product
  1 egg
  ½ teaspoon salt or salt substitute
  ¼ teaspoon freshly ground black pepper
  ½ cup grated sharp Cheddar cheese

Place lentils, vegetable stock, and bay leaf in a small saucepan. Bring to a boil, reduce to a simmer, cover and cook for 30 minutes, until lentils are tender. Drain and remove bay leaf.

In a medium saucepan, heat olive oil over medium heat. Add onion slices and garlic and cook, stirring frequently, for 3 to 4 minutes.

(continued)

Moussaka (continued)

Add mushrooms and cook for another 3 minutes. Stir in cooked lentils, tomatoes, tomato paste, and herbs. Bring to a boil, reduce heat, and simmer for 10 minutes. It should be thick and almost dry.

Meanwhile, preheat the broiler.

Slice unpeeled eggplant into ½-inch-thick slices crosswise, then cut slices in half. Spray both sides with olive oil spray.

Place eggplant slices on broiler pan or a cookie sheet and cook, about 4 inches from heating element, 3 to 4 minutes on each side, or until golden brown.

Preheat the oven to 350 degrees F. Spray a large shallow 9-by-13-inch baking pan with olive oil spray.

Mix yogurt with egg whites, egg, salt, and pepper in a medium bowl and beat well.

Layer half the eggplant in two rows down the length of the pan, overlapping pieces slightly. Pour lentil-tomato mixture evenly over eggplant. Arrange remaining eggplant on top, in two rows of overlapping pieces. Pour yogurt mixture evenly into the baking pan.

Bake for 30 minutes, sprinkle Cheddar cheese on top, and bake 15 more minutes until top is golden brown and bubbly. If the top isn't nicely browned, preheat broiler and brown for 1 minute until golden.

PER SERVING: 233 calories; 6 g fat (21.4% calories from fat); 18 g protein; 29 g carbohydrate; 12 g dietary fiber; 78 mg cholesterol; 304 mg sodium. EXCHANGES: 1 grain (starch); 1½ lean meat; 1½ vegetable; ½ fat.

Mushroom Madness

A delightful mélange of mushrooms and tofu.

MAKES 6 SERVINGS   PREPARATION TIME: 25 MINUTES

1   *teaspoon sesame oil*
2   *teaspoons plus 1 tablespoon low-sodium soy sauce*
⅛   *teaspoon red pepper flakes*
1   *(14-ounce) package firm tofu, drained and cut into ¾-inch cubes*
6   *tablespoons low-sodium vegetable broth*
1   *tablespoon dry sherry*
1   *tablespoon hoisin sauce (optional)*
1   *teaspoon cornstarch*
1   *tablespoon cold water*
2   *teaspoons hazelnut oil or extra-virgin olive oil*
2   *cloves garlic, peeled and minced*
1   *teaspoon grated gingerroot or ½ teaspoon ground ginger*
3   *cups mushrooms (a combination of white and brown plus exotic varieties, preferably straw and shiitake)*
3   *cups cooked rice (long-grain brown or basmati)*
2   *green onions, shredded*

Combine sesame oil, 2 teaspoons soy sauce, and pepper flakes in a medium container with a tight-fitting lid. Add tofu, place lid on securely, and shake to evenly coat tofu. Marinate for 10 minutes, shaking and inverting container 2 to 3 times. Remove from marinade and drain.

Mix broth, sherry, 1 tablespoon soy sauce, and hoisin sauce in a small bowl and set aside. Mix cornstarch and water together in another small bowl.

(continued)

Mushroom Madness *(continued)*

Heat 1 teaspoon oil in a nonstick wok or large skillet over high heat. Add garlic and ginger and stir-fry for 15 seconds. Add tofu to the wok and continue to cook, stirring often, for 3 to 4 minutes. Remove from pan.

Add remaining teaspoon of oil to the wok. Add mushrooms and stir-fry for 3 minutes. Pour in sherry mixture, turn down heat, and simmer for 4 to 5 minutes, stirring occasionally.

Pour cornstarch mixture into the wok and cook, stirring constantly, until sauce has thickened. Transfer tofu to the wok and toss gently. Turn heat up to medium and cook until heated through, about 3 minutes.

Serve over rice (½ cup per serving) and garnish with shredded green onions.

PER SERVING: 219 calories; 6 g fat (23.4% calories from fat); 10 g protein; 32 g carbohydrate; 1 g dietary fiber; trace cholesterol; 252 mg sodium. EXCHANGES: 2 grain (starch); 1½ lean meat; ½ vegetable; 1 fat.

SERVING IDEAS: Serve this with Mandarin Salad (page 131) and Sesame Green Beans (page 256). This dish may also be "greened up" by stir-frying ½ pound asparagus, zucchini, broccoli, or another green vegetable along with the mushrooms.

Note

Hoisin sauce, a thick, dark, spicy-sweet sauce made from garlic, soybeans, chiles, and other spices, is a classic accompaniment to moo shoo. It's a bit of an acquired taste, so give it a try before adding it to a dish. You'll find it in ethnic stores and in the gourmet section of supermarkets.

Curried Vegetables with Tofu

Tofu takes on an Indian flavor in this one-dish meal.

MAKES 4 SERVINGS   PREPARATION TIME: 40 MINUTES

1½ cups low-sodium vegetable broth or chicken broth
¾ cup quinoa
Olive oil spray
½ (14-ounce) package firm tofu cut into ½-inch cubes
1 teaspoon extra-virgin olive oil
1 medium onion, cut into ½-inch cubes
1 red bell pepper, cored and diced into ½-inch pieces
2 cups sliced white or brown mushrooms
1 teaspoon turmeric
1 teaspoon ground cumin
1 teaspoon ground coriander
Dash cayenne pepper, or to taste
1 cup frozen peas, thawed
1 tablespoon low-sodium soy sauce

Bring broth to a boil in a medium saucepan. Rinse quinoa well, add to saucepan, and reduce heat, and simmer until liquid has been absorbed, about 15 minutes.

Heat a large nonstick skillet over medium heat and spray it with olive oil spray. Pat tofu dry with paper towels and add to the skillet. Cook, tossing often, until golden brown, about 5 minutes. Remove from the skillet and keep warm.

(continued)

Curried Vegetables with Tofu (*continued*)

Pour olive oil into skillet, heat over medium heat, then add onion, red pepper, and mushrooms. Cook for 5 minutes, stirring often, until onion and pepper are tender-crisp. Add all of the spices, (or 1 tablespoon curry powder), and cook, stirring constantly, for 1 minute.

Add tofu, peas, quinoa, and soy sauce to the skillet and cook, gently tossing, until piping hot. Serve immediately.

PER SERVING: 248 calories; 7 g fat (23.8% calories from fat); 16 g protein; 34 g carbohydrate; 7 g dietary fiber; 398 mg sodium. EXCHANGES: 2 grain (starch); 1½ lean meat; ½ vegetable; 1 fat.

SERVING IDEAS: Serve this with Raita (page 286) and a green salad. It is also good chilled.

Note

You may use 1 tablespoon curry powder instead of the spices, if desired. When you're cooking with curry, turn on the fan and open the windows. The odor of curry can linger for days.

Zen Stir-Fry

A simple but delicious stir-fry.

2¼ cups water
¾ cup pearl barley
1½ teaspoons extra-virgin olive oil
2 large carrots, cut into ½-inch pieces
1 large onion, cut into ½-inch wedges
2 cloves garlic, peeled and minced
1 medium zucchini, cut into ½-inch pieces
8 ounces white or brown mushrooms, halved
6 cups fresh spinach, stems removed and cleaned, or 10-ounce bag cleaned spinach
1½ tablespoons low-sodium soy sauce

Bring water to a boil, add barley, lower heat, cover, and cook for 45 minutes, until barley is barely tender and water has evaporated.

Ten minutes before barley is ready, heat ½ teaspoon olive oil in a large nonstick skillet or wok over medium-high heat. Add carrots and sauté, stirring often, for 3 minutes. Add another ½ teaspoon olive oil and onion to the skillet and sauté for another 3 minutes. Add remaining ½ teaspoon olive oil, garlic, zucchini, and mushrooms and continue cooking and stirring for 3 more minutes. Add spinach and soy sauce and continue to cook, stirring constantly, for 1 to 2 minutes, until spinach wilts.

Serve over hot barley.

(continued)

Zen Stir-Fry (continued)

PER SERVING: 224 calories; 4 g fat (16.5% calories from fat); 8 g protein; 42 g carbohydrate; 10 g dietary fiber; 0 mg cholesterol; 285 mg sodium. EXCHANGES: 2 grain (starch); 2½ vegetable; ½ fat.

SERVING IDEA: This is also nice over cooked quinoa, wheat, and other whole grains. (Limit grain to ½ cup per serving.)

Note
Of all the whole grains, rice is the most problematic for diabetics, for it has a high glycemic index and is therefore likely to drive up blood sugar levels. Long-grain brown rice and basmati rice have less of an adverse effect than other types of rice. Cooking rice until just tender will also help. Finally, eat rice in moderation—no more than ½ cup per serving—or substitute with lower-glycemic grains, such as barley, quinoa, and bulgur.

Moo Shoo Vegetables in Lettuce Leaves

Romaine leaves make this dish a snap.

MAKES 4 SERVINGS   PREPARATION TIME: 40 MINUTES

1   head romaine lettuce
1   tablespoon rice wine or dry sherry
1   tablespoon low-sodium soy sauce
1   teaspoon xylitol or honey
1   teaspoon cornstarch
⅓   cup water
    Olive oil spray
8   egg whites or 1 cup Egg Beaters or other egg white product
1   teaspoon hazelnut oil or olive oil
2   teaspoons grated gingerroot or 1 teaspoon ground ginger
2   cups finely shredded cabbage
1   large carrot, shredded
6   green onions (with green tops), cut lengthwise into thin shreds
2   cups mushrooms, thinly sliced
½   cup canned bamboo shoots, drained and cut lengthwise into thin
    strips
½   cup canned water chestnuts, finely chopped
¼   cup hoisin sauce or Mandarin Dipping Sauce (page 291)

Remove base from romaine and separate leaves, discarding dam-
aged outer leaves. Wash, dry, and set aside.

In a small bowl, combine rice wine, soy sauce, xylitol, cornstarch,
and water. Set aside.

(continued)

Moo Shoo Vegetables in Lettuce Leaves *(continued)*

Spray a medium nonstick skillet with olive oil spray and heat over medium heat. Add egg whites and cook like an omelet, lifting edges and allowing uncooked egg to run underneath. Cook until set, about 3 minutes. Remove from the skillet and cut into thin strips.

In a large nonstick wok or skillet, heat oil over medium heat. Add the ginger and stir-fry for 15 seconds. Add cabbage, carrot, and onions and stir-fry for 2 minutes. Add mushrooms and stir-fry for 2 more minutes. Add bamboo shoots, water chestnuts, and cooked egg, and continue to stir-fry for 2 more minutes. Stir in the soy sauce–cornstarch mixture and cook, stirring, as sauce thickens, another 2 minutes. Transfer to a serving bowl.

Serve with romaine leaves and hoisin sauce or Mandarin Dipping Sauce.

PER SERVING (not including sauce): 131 calories; 2 g fat (12.4% calories from fat); 13 g protein; 18 g carbohydrate; 7 g dietary fiber; 0 mg cholesterol; 298 mg sodium. EXCHANGES: 1 lean meat; 3 vegetable.

SERVING IDEAS: Diners take a romaine leaf, spoon moo shoo vegetables into it, fold or roll it up, and dip it in the sauces. Messy but fun! Moo shoo may also be served over rice or noodles.

Note
Traditional moo shoo is spooned into crepelike pancakes. We think you'll like this version with romaine leaves.

Stuffed Portobello Mushrooms

Pesto gives these mushrooms a wonderfully intense flavor.

MAKES 4 SERVINGS   PREPARATION TIME: 40 MINUTES

- 4 large (5- to 6-inch) portobello mushrooms
  Olive oil spray
- 3 green onions, thinly sliced
- 1 cup finely chopped zucchini
- ¾ cup finely chopped carrots
- ¼ teaspoon Low-Sodium Seasoned Salt (page 297) or salt substitute
- ⅛ teaspoon freshly ground black pepper
- 4 tablespoons Pesto (page 296) or store-bought pesto
- 3 tablespoons bread crumbs (preferably sprouted-grain)
- ¼ cup grated part skim milk mozzarella cheese
- 8 fresh basil leaves

Remove stems from mushrooms and chop.

Preheat the oven to 425 degrees F. Spray a baking sheet with olive oil spray.

Spray a large nonstick skillet with olive oil spray and heat over medium heat. Add chopped mushroom stems, green onions, zucchini, carrots, salt, and pepper and sauté, stirring occasionally, until tender-crisp, 3 to 4 minutes. Remove from the heat, and stir in pesto and bread crumbs.

Spoon mixture into mushroom caps and place mushrooms on baking sheet. Bake until mushrooms are tender, about 15 minutes. Sprinkle cheese over mushrooms and cook for another 3 minutes, or until cheese melts.

Garnish with basil leaves.

(continued)

Stuffed Portobello Mushrooms *(continued)*

PER SERVING (includes pesto): 173 calories; 9 g fat (45.0% calories from fat); 9 g protein; 16 g carbohydrate; 4 g dietary fiber; 8 mg cholesterol; 287 mg sodium. EXCHANGES: ½ lean meat; 2½ vegetable; 1½ fat.

SERVING IDEAS: This may also be served as an appetizer. Slice the mushrooms into 1-inch wedges, and garnish the serving plate with fresh basil leaves.

Note

Large portobello mushroom caps can be stuffed with anything. These are some variations:

Spinach-cheese: Replace zucchini and carrots with 2 cups fresh or ¾ cup frozen spinach. Replace pesto with 4 tablespoons feta cheese.

Shrimp: Replace carrots with ½ cup small, cooked shrimp and add 2 cloves minced garlic. Replace pesto with 4 tablespoons spaghetti or tomato sauce.

Olive: Replace pesto with 4 tablespoons Black Olive Tapenade (page 66).

Stuffed Peppers Provençale

Full of the flavors of the South of France.

MAKES 4 SERVINGS   PREPARATION TIME: 1 HOUR

2 *extra large bell peppers (green, red, or yellow)*
  Olive oil spray
1 *teaspoon extra-virgin olive oil*
1 *clove garlic, peeled and minced*
1 *medium onion, thinly sliced*
1 *small zucchini, thinly sliced*
1 *cup thinly sliced mushrooms*
1 *(14½-ounce) can low-sodium tomatoes with juice, coarsely chopped*
1 *cup canned white beans (or other beans), rinsed and drained*
1 *tablespoon tomato paste*
1 *tablespoon freshly chopped basil or 1 teaspoon dried basil*
¼ *teaspoon salt or salt substitute*
⅛ *teaspoon freshly ground black pepper*
4 *tablespoons grated Parmesan cheese*

Bring 6 cups of water to a boil in a large saucepan.

Meanwhile, cut peppers in half lengthwise through stems. Remove stems, seeds, and membranes. Blanch peppers in boiling water for 3 minutes. Drain and set aside.

Preheat the oven to 350 degrees F. Spray a medium-sized shallow baking pan with olive oil spray.

Stuffed Peppers Provençale (continued)

Heat olive oil in a large skillet over medium heat. Add garlic, onion, and zucchini and sauté, stirring often, for 5 minutes. Add mushrooms and continue to sauté, stirring often, for 3 more minutes. Add tomatoes, beans, and tomato paste and bring to a boil. Cook uncovered for 5 to 8 minutes, stirring occasionally, until liquid evaporates. Remove from the heat and stir in basil, salt, and pepper.

Fill bell peppers with vegetable mixture and place in the prepared baking pan. Cover with aluminum foil and bake 20 minutes. Remove foil and sprinkle 1 tablespoon Parmesan cheese over each stuffed pepper. Return to the oven and continue baking for 5 to 10 more minutes, until heated through.

PER SERVING: 157 calories; 3 g fat (17.3% calories from fat); 9 g protein; 25 g carbohydrate; 6 g dietary fiber; 4 mg cholesterol; 418 mg sodium. EXCHANGES: 1 grain (starch); ½ lean meat; 2½ vegetable; ½ fat.

Note

Many recipes call for just a spoonful or two of tomato paste. Store leftover tomato paste in tablespoon-sized portions wrapped in plastic wrap in a bag in the freezer for future use.

Springtime Frittata

Who says eggs are only served for breakfast?

MAKES 4 SERVINGS   PREPARATION TIME: 25 MINUTES

¾ *pound asparagus*
12 *egg whites or 1½ cups Egg Beaters or other egg white product*
4 *tablespoons grated Parmesan cheese*
1 *teaspoon extra-virgin olive oil*
1 *bunch green onions, sliced*
2 *tablespoons low-sodium chicken broth*
¼ *teaspoon freshly ground black pepper*
2 *tablespoons freshly chopped chives, for garnish*

Snap tough stems off asparagus. Leave an inch or so of tips whole, and cut stems into ½-inch slices.

In a medium bowl, stir egg whites and cheese until well blended.

In a large nonstick covered skillet, heat olive oil over medium heat. Add green onions and cook, stirring constantly, for 1 minute. Add asparagus, broth, and pepper to the skillet. Stir, cover, lower heat, and cook for 2 to 3 minutes, until asparagus is tender-crisp. Remove cover, turn heat up to medium, and cook for another minute or so until broth has evaporated.

Preheat the broiler.

Spread vegetables evenly over the bottom of the skillet. Pour in egg mixture and shake the skillet to distribute evenly. Reduce heat to low, cover, and cook for 3 to 5 minutes, without stirring, until eggs begin to set at edges.

(continued)

Springtime Frittata (continued)

Remove cover. Use a spatula to lift up edge of eggs. The bottom should be nicely browned. The top will still be runny. If bottom isn't browned, turn heat to medium and cook a couple of minutes longer.

Place the skillet under the broiler, the handle sticking out of the oven, for 2 to 4 minutes, until the eggs are set, puffy, and beginning to brown. Be careful when you remove the skillet from the oven. The handle will be very hot!

Slide frittata out of the skillet onto a serving plate and garnish with chives. Cut into wedges.

PER SERVING: 96 calories; 3 g fat (26.2% calories from fat); 14 g protein; 4 g carbohydrate; 1 g dietary fiber; 4 mg cholesterol; 260 mg sodium. EXCHANGES: 1½ lean meat; ½ vegetable; ½ fat.

Note
Asparagus can be replaced with chopped zucchini, green peppers, onions, mushrooms, spinach, broccoli, or any combination of vegetables.

Mexican Pizza

Pizza with a Mexican flair.

MAKES 4 SERVINGS   PREPARATION TIME: 25 MINUTES

4 *whole wheat tortillas*
1 *(15-ounce) can fat-free refried beans*
½ *cup grated low-sodium Cheddar cheese*
½ *cup chopped green onions*
1 *large tomato, chopped*
4 *tablespoons sliced ripe olives*
2 *cups shredded lettuce*
½ *cup freshly chopped cilantro*

Preheat the oven to 350 degrees F.

Place tortillas on an ungreased cookie sheet and bake for 5 minutes. Cool for a few minutes.

Handling gently (they'll be crisp), turn tortillas over and spread the refried beans, evenly divided, on each. Top with cheese.

Return to the oven and bake for another 5 minutes, until beans are warm and cheese melts.

Top with green onions, tomato, olives, lettuce, and cilantro. Cut into quarters for easier eating.

PER SERVING: 185 calories; 6 g fat (26% calories from fat); 9 g protein; 30 g carbohydrate; 2 g dietary fiber; 14 mg cholesterol; 369 mg sodium. EXCHANGES: 2 grain (starch); ½ lean meat; ½ vegetable; 1 fat.

(continued)

Mexican Pizza (continued)

SERVING IDEAS: Serve with Mary's Fresh Salsa (page 283) or Quick and Easy Salsa (page 284) or your favorite low-sodium brand. For an even heartier meal, place up to ¼ cup of cooked, chopped chicken on top of the beans before cooking. Mexican Pizza may also be cut into eighths and served as an appetizer.

Note
You can create a lower-carb Italian pizza by preparing tortillas as described in this recipe, then topping them with tomato sauce, mushrooms, mozzarella cheese, and your other favorite pizza toppings.

Side Dishes

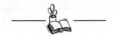

According to the United States Department of Agriculture's latest "What We Eat in America" survey, the average American eats only one serving of whole-grain foods and three servings of vegetables a day. This is unfortunate, for these foods are our most abundant sources of vitamins, minerals, fiber, and phytonutrients, which all offer a vast array of health benefits.

You can step head and shoulders above the average by adding side dishes of vegetables and whole grains to your meals. They can be as simple as cooking your favorite vegetables for a few minutes in a steamer or microwave and boiling up a pot of seasoned barley or another whole grain. Or you can soar above the average by incorporating the delicious recipes in this chapter into your repertoire. We've included the most nutrient-dense vegetables (Louisiana-Style Greens, page 252, and Broccoli with Lemon-Chive Sauce, page 260) and heartiest low-glycemic grains (Quinoa Pilaf, page 268, and Wild Rice and Mushroom Medley, page 264), as well as healthy versions of everyone's all-time favorite side dishes (Sweet Potato "Fries," page 263, and Pecan Stuffing, page 269).

Plan your side dishes to complement your main course. If you're preparing a protein-rich dish of grilled fish or sautéed chicken breast, make sure your sides contain whole grains and green vegetables. On the other hand, if your entrée is pasta or otherwise carbohydrate-heavy, complement it with vegetables and/or salad.

Louisiana-Style Greens

Loaded with potassium, vitamin A, and folate.

MAKES 4 SERVINGS   PREPARATION TIME: 50 MINUTES

1 *pound greens (mustard, turnip, collards, or a combination)*
1 *clove garlic, peeled and minced*
1 *medium onion, chopped*
2 *cups low-sodium chicken broth*
½ *teaspoon freshly ground black pepper*
¼ *teaspoon salt or salt substitute*

Wash greens carefully and remove tough stems.

Place all ingredients in a large saucepan or stockpot. Bring to a boil over medium heat. Reduce heat and cook, stirring occasionally, for 35 minutes, or until tender. Drain and serve.

PER SERVING: 57 calories; 2 g fat (15.8% calories from fat); 9 g protein; 9 g carbohydrate; 4 g dietary fiber; 0 mg cholesterol; 183 mg sodium. EXCHANGES: ½ lean meat; 1½ vegetable.

Note
Mustard, turnip, collard, and other leafy greens are extremely rich in vitamins, minerals, and protective phytonutrients. They are also very dirty. To save time, look for prewashed, packaged fresh or frozen greens.

Grilled Pesto Vegetables

A great way to prepare summer's bounty.

MAKES 4 SERVINGS   PREPARATION TIME: 25 MINUTES

2 *medium zucchini*
1 *small eggplant*
12 *large white or brown mushrooms or 4 medium portobello*
   mushrooms
   Olive oil spray
½ *cup Pesto (page 296) or store-bought pesto*

Preheat the grill or broiler and place the grill or broiler pan 3 to 4 inches from heat.

Prepare vegetables as follows: slice zucchini lengthwise into ½-inch slices; peel eggplant and slice crosswise into ½-inch slices; remove stems and clean mushrooms.

Spray the grill with olive oil spray. Spray both sides of vegetables with olive oil spray.

Place vegetables on the grill (mushroom caps facing down) and cook 5 minutes. Turn and continue cooking 3 to 5 minutes.

Remove from the grill and brush vegetable slices with Pesto.

PER SERVING (includes Pesto): 209 calories; 15 g fat (59.1% calories from fat); 8 g protein; 14 g carbohydrate; 5 g dietary fiber; 9 mg cholesterol; 215 mg sodium. EXCHANGES: ½ lean meat; 2½ vegetable; 2½ fat.

Note
Everybody grills burgers and chicken, but many people don't think to prepare vegetables in this way. It's quick, easy, and delicious, especially when paired with fragrant basil-infused pesto.

Garlicky Spinach
A bold way to liven up spinach.

MAKES 4 SERVINGS   PREPARATION TIME: 15 MINUTES

8 cups (1 large bunch) fresh spinach
1 teaspoon extra-virgin olive oil
2 cloves garlic, peeled and minced

Wash spinach well and remove tough stems.

In a large nonstick skillet, heat olive oil over medium-high heat.

Add minced garlic and cook, stirring for 1 minute.

Add spinach to the skillet and cook, stirring constantly and pushing uncooked spinach toward the bottom of the skillet. Cook until all spinach has wilted, 3 to 4 minutes.

PER SERVING: 25 calories; 1 g fat (40.5% calories from fat); 2 g protein; 3 g carbohydrate; 2 g dietary fiber; 0 mg cholesterol; 48 mg sodium. EXCHANGE: ½ vegetable.

SERVING IDEA: Garlicky Spinach makes a nice bed for a fillet of fish or a chicken breast.

Note
Garlic contains sulfur compounds that have numerous health benefits. It lowers cholesterol, reduces blood pressure, fights infections, and inhibits the growth of some cancer cells.

Stir-Fried Asparagus

Enjoy this in the spring when fresh asparagus is in season.

MAKES 4 SERVINGS   PREPARATION TIME: 20 MINUTES

1 *pound asparagus*
2 *teaspoons hoisin sauce, optional (see Note on page 236)*
2 *teaspoons low-sodium soy sauce*
2 *tablespoons water*
  Dash red pepper flakes
1 *teaspoon hazelnut oil or almond oil or olive oil*
1 *medium onion, sliced lengthwise into ½-inch wedges*

Snap tough ends off asparagus. Cut asparagus spears into 1-inch pieces.

Combine hoisin sauce, soy sauce, water, and red pepper flakes in a small bowl.

Heat oil in a large nonstick skillet or wok over medium heat. Add onion slices and stir-fry for 2 minutes. Add asparagus to the skillet and stir-fry for 2 minutes.

Pour sauce into the skillet and cook 3 to 4 minutes, until asparagus is tender yet crisp.

PER SERVING: 42 calories; 1 g fat (27% calories from fat); 2 g protein; 7 g carbohydrate; 2 g dietary fiber; trace cholesterol; 145 mg sodium. EXCHANGES: 1 vegetable.

SERVING IDEAS: Good with any kind of Asian main dishes. This recipe works well with broccoli, green beans, and other vegetables.

Sesame Green Beans

Good served hot or cold.

MAKES 4 SERVINGS   PREPARATION TIME: 20 MINUTES

1 *pound fresh green beans*
2 *teaspoons sesame oil*
1 *tablespoon low-sodium soy sauce*
⅛ *teaspoon red pepper flakes*
1 *tablespoon sesame seeds, for garnish*

Snip ends off beans.

Bring 1 inch water to boil in a large saucepan. Add beans and boil, uncovered, for 5 minutes. Cover, reduce heat, and boil another 5 minutes until beans are tender, yet still crisp.

Meanwhile, mix sesame oil, soy sauce, and red pepper flakes in a small bowl.

When beans are done, transfer to a serving bowl, toss with sesame oil–soy sauce mixture, and top with sesame seeds.

PER SERVING: 66 calories; 4 g fat (42.9% calories from fat); 2 g protein; 8 g carbohydrate; 4 g dietary fiber; 0 mg cholesterol; 156 mg sodium. EXCHANGES: 1½ vegetable; ½ fat.

SERVING IDEA: These may also be refrigerated and served cold. They go well with Teriyaki Salmon (page 198).

Note

Sesame oil has more polyunsaturated fats than the other oils we recommend for cooking. This means it doesn't tolerate heat as well, so add it at the end, after cooking and just before serving.

Roasted Winter Vegetables

This hearty dish is redolent of rosemary.

MAKES 4 SERVINGS   PREPARATION TIME: 1 HOUR

2 *medium carrots*
2 *large leeks*
2 *medium onions*
2 *small sweet potatoes, peeled*
1 *tablespoon extra-virgin olive oil*
2 *cloves garlic, peeled and minced*
1 *sprig rosemary, chopped, or 1 teaspoon dried rosemary*
½ *teaspoon salt or salt substitute*
¼ *teaspoon freshly ground black pepper*
2 *tablespoons balsamic vinegar*

Preheat the oven to 400 degrees F.

Peel and trim vegetables and prepare as follows: cut carrots and leeks into 1-inch pieces, onions into eighths, and sweet potatoes into 1-inch cubes.

Mix olive oil with garlic, rosemary, salt, and pepper.

Place vegetables in a shallow 9-by-13-inch pan. Pour olive oil mixture over vegetables and mix well, coating evenly.

Roast, uncovered, for 40 to 50 minutes, or until vegetables are tender and lightly browned.

Transfer to a serving dish and sprinkle with balsamic vinegar.

PER SERVING: 168 calories; 4 g fat (20.4% calories from fat); 3 g protein; 32 g carbohydrate; 5 g dietary fiber; 0 mg cholesterol; 299 mg sodium. EXCHANGES: 1 grain (starch); 3 vegetable; ½ fat.

(continued)

Roasted Winter Vegetables *(continued)*

SERVING IDEA: All you need is a piece of broiled or lightly sautéed chicken or fish for a complete meal.

Note

Traditional balsamic vinegar comes from Modena, Italy. Made from the grapes grown in the area, it is fermented in wooden barrels for a minimum of twelve years. The finished product, which may cost as much as fine cognac, is dark, thick, resinlike, and aromatic. Less expensive balsamic vinegar, labeled "unaged" and fermented only for several months, isn't bad, but spending a little more for aged balsamic is definitely worth it.

Zucchini-Leek Sauté

Overrun with garden zucchini? Try this simple, delicious recipe.

MAKES 4 SERVINGS　　　　　　　　　PREPARATION TIME: 15 MINUTES

2 *medium leeks*
1 *teaspoon extra-virgin olive oil*
4 *small zucchini, cut into ¼- to ½-inch slices (4 cups total)*
¼ *teaspoon Low-Sodium Seasoned Salt (page 297) or salt substitute*
2 *tablespoons grated Parmesan cheese*
1 *tablespoon freshly chopped basil (optional)*

Trim green ends off leeks, then slice white parts into ¼- to ½-inch slices.

Heat olive oil over medium-high heat in a large nonstick skillet.

Add zucchini, leeks, and salt and cook, stirring frequently until just tender, about 3 to 5 minutes. Remove from heat and stir in Parmesan cheese and basil.

PER SERVING: 79 calories; 2 g fat (23.6% calories from fat); 4 g protein; 13 g carbohydrate; 4 g dietary fiber; 2 mg cholesterol; 147 mg sodium. EXCHANGES: 2 vegetable; ½ fat.

Note
Parsley, tarragon, or another favorite herb may be used in place of basil.

Broccoli with Lemon-Chive Sauce

Nutrient-rich broccoli with a healthy alternative to cheese sauce.

MAKES 4 SERVINGS   PREPARATION TIME: 15 MINUTES

4 *cups broccoli florets*
½ *cup Lemon-Chive Sauce (page 288)*

Steam broccoli over boiling water for 5 to 7 minutes, until tender-crisp. (Or place in a covered glass dish with 2 tablespoons of water and cook in the microwave for 2 to 3 minutes.)

Pour Lemon-Chive Sauce over hot broccoli and serve.

PER SERVING (includes Lemon-Chive Sauce): 44 calories; 1 g fat (23.2% calories from fat); 3 g protein; 6 g carbohydrate; 2 g dietary fiber; 3 mg cholesterol; 120 mg sodium. EXCHANGE: ½ vegetable.

Note
If broccoli tastes bitter to you, maybe you're a "super taster." Super tasters, who make up about 25 percent of the population, have more than the average amount of taste buds. Another 25 percent have fewer than average.

Artichokes with Healthy Hollandaise Sauce

Kids love the drama of eating artichokes.

MAKES 4 SERVINGS   PREPARATION TIME: 1 HOUR

4 *artichokes*
½ *lemon*
¾ *cup Healthy Hollandaise Sauce (page 289)*

Wash artichokes, cut off stems at base, and remove small bottom and tough outer leaves. Cut about 2 inches off top of each artichoke, then trim sharp tips off ends of outer leaves with kitchen shears or scissors. Rub cut edges with lemon.

Stand artichokes upright in a deep saucepan large enough to hold snugly. Fill saucepan one-third full with water. Bring to a boil and adjust heat to maintain water at a gentle boil. Cover and cook for 30 to 45 minutes, depending on size, until base can be pierced easily with a fork and insides of leaves are tender. Add a little more boiling water, if needed. Turn artichokes upside down to drain.

Serve on individual plates with a small dish of Healthy Hollandaise Sauce for each person.

PER SERVING (includes Healthy Hollandaise Sauce): 113 calories; 2 g fat (16% calories from fat); 6 g protein; 20 g carbohydrate; 7 g dietary fiber; 56 mg cholesterol; 287 mg sodium. EXCHANGE: 2½ vegetable.

(continued)

Artichokes with Healthy Hollandiase Sauce *(continued)*

SERVING IDEAS: Instead of serving hot with Healthy Hollandaise Sauce, serve cold with Basic Vinaigrette (page 274) or Homemade Mayonnaise (page 279). To eat, pull a leaf off, dip the base into some sauce, and pull the leaf through your teeth to remove the soft inner pulp. When you get to the fuzzy center, scrape it out and discard it. The remaining heart is considered to be the best part of the artichoke. Provide a large bowl (or individual bowls) for discarded leaves. Whoever misses the bowl has to do the dishes.

Sweet Potato "Fries"

These oven-baked fries sidestep the excessive calories,
transfats, and high glycemic index of regular fries.

MAKES 4 SERVINGS   PREPARATION TIME: 40 MINUTES

Olive oil spray
2 *medium sweet potatoes*
2 *tablespoons extra-virgin olive oil*
1 *teaspoon garlic powder*
1 *teaspoon onion powder*
½ *teaspoon Low-Sodium Seasoned Salt (page 297) or salt substitute*
½ *teaspoon freshly ground black pepper*

Preheat the oven to 400 degrees F. Spray a baking sheet with olive oil spray.

Peel sweet potatoes and cut into ½-inch sticks.

Combine olive oil and spices in a large bowl. Toss potato sticks in oil until evenly coated.

Arrange potato sticks in a single layer on the baking sheet. Bake for 25 to 30 minutes, until golden brown and tender. Flip with a spatula after 15 minutes to prevent sticking.

PER SERVING: 133 calories; 7 g fat (46.2% calories from fat); 1 g protein; 17 g carbohydrate; 2 g dietary fiber; 0 mg cholesterol; 180 mg sodium. EXCHANGES: 1 grain (starch); 1½ fat.

Note

Confused about sweet potatoes and yams? Join the club. The orange, moist, dark-skinned varieties commonly referred to as yams and the pale, drier sweet potatoes are both, in fact, sweet potatoes. True yams are a completely different species and are rarely sold in North American supermarkets. Pale, dry sweet potatoes work best in this recipe.

Wild Rice and Mushroom Medley

*The crunchy bite of wild rice complements the
earthy flavor of mushrooms.*

MAKES 5 SERVINGS   PREPARATION TIME: 1 HOUR 15 MINUTES

2⅓ cups low-sodium chicken broth
 1 cup wild rice
 1 teaspoon extra-virgin olive oil
 1 medium onion, chopped
 8 ounces mushrooms, sliced (about 4 cups) (See Note)
 ½ teaspoon poultry seasoning

Bring broth to a boil in a medium saucepan with a tight-fitting lid.
Add wild rice, return to a boil, reduce heat, cover and simmer 45 to
50 minutes, or until rice is tender and kernels begin to burst open.
Let sit covered for 10 minutes. Fluff with a fork and drain any
excess liquid.

In a large nonstick skillet, heat olive oil over medium heat. Add
onion and sauté for 3 minutes. Add mushrooms and seasoning and
cook, stirring occasionally, for another 3 to 5 minutes.

Gently stir in wild rice and cook until heated through, about
3 minutes.

PER SERVING: 165 calories; 1 g fat (7.6% calories from fat); 11 g protein; 29 g carbohydrate; 3 g dietary fiber; 0 mg cholesterol; 246 mg
sodium. EXCHANGES: 1½ grain (starch); ½ lean meat; 1 vegetable;
1 fat.

SERVING IDEA: Serve this with any fish or poultry dish.

Note

Experiment with exotic mushrooms such as shiitake, oyster, and straw mushrooms. They each have their own distinctive shapes and flavors and really enhance this dish.

Garbanzo Curry

*Curry contains turmeric, one of nature's
most powerful anti-inflammatories.*

MAKES 4 SERVINGS   PREPARATION TIME: 40 MINUTES

1 cup dried garbanzo beans or 2 cups canned garbanzo beans,
   drained and rinsed
2 teaspoons extra-virgin olive oil
1 tablespoon curry powder
1 onion, chopped
1 cup water
2 cups Swiss chard leaves, beet greens, spinach, or other greens,
   tightly packed, or 10-ounce package frozen chopped spinach
1 tomato
¼ teaspoon salt or salt substitute

If using dried beans, soak 1 cup garbanzos overnight, drain, rinse well, and place in a medium saucepan. Cover with water, and bring to a boil over high heat. Reduce heat, cover, and simmer 1½ to 2 hours, or until tender, adding additional water as needed to keep beans just covered. Drain before using.

Heat olive oil over medium heat in a large saucepan, stockpot, or Dutch oven. Add curry powder and stir constantly for 30 to 45 seconds.

Add onion to the saucepan and cook for 2 minutes, stirring frequently.

Add cooked garbanzos and water to the saucepan. Bring to a boil, reduce heat, and simmer, uncovered, for 30 minutes, adding more water as necessary.

Meanwhile, coarsely chop greens and tomato. Add to the saucepan, along with salt. Continue cooking over low heat until greens are tender, 5 to 10 minutes.

PER SERVING: 185 calories; 5 g fat (23.1% calories from fat); 9 g protein; 29 g carbohydrate; 5 g dietary fiber; 0 mg cholesterol; 177 mg sodium. EXCHANGES: 1½ grain (starch); ½ lean meat; 1 vegetable; ½ fat.

SERVING IDEA: Serve this with one of the simple grilled or baked fish or chicken dishes, with Raita (page 286) on the side.

Quinoa Pilaf

Quinoa—a grain you must get acquainted with.

MAKES 4 SERVINGS   PREPARATION TIME: 35 MINUTES

1 *teaspoon extra-virgin olive oil*
½ *cup finely chopped carrot*
½ *cup finely chopped celery*
½ *cup finely chopped onion*
1 *clove garlic, peeled and minced*
¾ *cup quinoa*
1½ *cups low-sodium chicken broth*

Heat olive oil in a medium saucepan over medium heat. Add carrot, celery, onion, and garlic and sauté, stirring frequently, for 3 minutes.

Rinse quinoa well and drain. Add to saucepan and cook, stirring, for 3 to 4 minutes.

Add the chicken broth and bring to a boil. Lower heat and simmer for about 20 minutes, or until liquid is absorbed.

Fluff with a fork and serve.

PER SERVING: 158 calories; 4 g fat (20.1% calories from fat); 9 g protein; 27 g carbohydrate; 3 g dietary fiber; 0 mg cholesterol; 41 mg sodium. EXCHANGES: 1½ grain (starch); ½ lean meat; 1 vegetable; ½ fat.

Note

Quinoa, which is native to Peru, is billed as the grain of the Inca empire. It has more protein than any other grain and contains all the essential amino acids. Another plus is that it cooks considerably faster than most other whole grains.

Pecan Stuffing

A stuffing made with sprouted-grain bread that
won't get a rise out of your blood sugar.

MAKES 6 SERVINGS   PREPARATION TIME: 1 HOUR

   6 *slices sprouted-grain bread*
   1 *teaspoon extra-virgin olive oil*
  ½ *cup chopped onion*
  ½ *cup chopped celery*
  ½ *cup chopped parsley, tightly packed*
  ¼ *cup coarsely chopped pecans*
   1 *teaspoon poultry seasoning*
1¼ *cups low-sodium chicken broth*
      Olive oil spray

Toast bread in a toaster. (Or toast all at once under the broiler, 1 to 2 minutes per side.) Cool and cut into small cubes.

Preheat the oven to 350 degrees F.

Heat olive oil in a large nonstick skillet over medium heat. Add onion and celery and cook until tender, about 3 minutes.

In a large bowl, combine bread cubes, onion and celery mixture, parsley, pecans, and poultry seasoning. Stir to blend well. Pour chicken broth into the bowl and stir until moistened.

Coat a medium baking dish with olive oil spray. Transfer stuffing to the baking dish, cover, and bake until hot, 30 to 40 minutes. (If you like a crispier top, remove the cover after 25 minutes.)

(continued)

Pecan Stuffing (continued)

PER SERVING: 136 calories; 4 g fat (28.1% calories from fat); 7 g protein; 18 g carbohydrate; 4 g dietary fiber; 0 mg cholesterol; 195 mg sodium. EXCHANGES: 1 grain (starch); 1 lean meat; ½ vegetable; ½ fat.

SERVING IDEA: Serve this with Gravy (page 293) as a side to roasted turkey, chicken, or other meat.

Note

You can also stuff a turkey or roasting chicken with Pecan Stuffing.

Moroccan Couscous
Exotic and tasty.

MAKES 4 SERVINGS · · · · · · · · · · · · PREPARATION TIME: 15 MINUTES

¾ cup low-sodium chicken broth
¾ cup couscous
1 tablespoon lemon juice
1 tablespoon extra-virgin olive oil
   Dash cinnamon
½ cup minced celery
¼ cup thinly sliced green onion
2 tablespoons minced parsley

Bring chicken broth to a boil in a 2-quart saucepan.

Stir couscous into boiling broth, remove from heat, and cover. Let stand 3 minutes.

Meanwhile, combine lemon juice, olive oil, and cinnamon and drizzle over couscous. Let stand another 3 minutes.

Remove lid, add celery, onion, and parsley and toss until mixed.

PER SERVING: 167 calories; 4 g fat (19.6% calories from fat); 7 g protein; 27 g carbohydrate; 2 g dietary fiber; 0 mg cholesterol; 115 mg sodium. EXCHANGES: 1½ grain (starch); ½ fat.

SERVING IDEAS: Serve warm or at room temperature with grilled fish or chicken, along with a green vegetable and salad.

Note
Couscous, like pasta, is made from hard durum wheat and therefore has a relatively low glycemic index.

Thai Noodles

Sesame oil gives these noodles an Asian flavor.

MAKES 4 SERVINGS   PREPARATION TIME: 30 MINUTES

5   *ounces linguine*
2   *tablespoons low-sodium soy sauce*
1   *tablespoon sesame oil*
⅛   *teaspoon red pepper flakes*
¼   *cup thinly sliced green onion*
1   *tablespoon freshly chopped cilantro*
1   *lime, quartered (optional)*

Cook linguine in boiling water per package directions, about 8 minutes, until al dente (just tender). Drain, rinse, and drain again.

Meanwhile, mix soy sauce, sesame oil, red pepper flakes, and green onion, stirring until well blended.

In a large skillet, toss cooked linguine and sauce together over medium heat until heated through.

Sprinkle cilantro over noodles and serve with lime wedges.

PER SERVING: 175 calories; 4 g fat (20.6% calories from fat); 5 g protein; 30 g carbohydrate; 1 g dietary fiber; 0 mg cholesterol; 305 mg sodium. EXCHANGES: 2 grain (starch); ½ vegetable; ½ fat.

SERVING IDEA: This is a nice summertime side dish with Grilled Shrimp Brochettes (page 213) or other grilled fish or poultry.

Sauces, Etc.

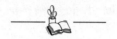

Woe to the cook whose sauce has no sting.
—Geoffrey Chaucer

The right sauce can elevate a mediocre dish to new heights. It can transform bland foods into succulent dishes and dress up the appearance of plain-looking dishes. We have included lots of recipes in this category: relishes, dipping sauces, seasoning mixes, spreads, fish and chicken toppers, salad dressings, gravies, and dessert sauces. It was a challenge to transform some of our favorite sauces from decadent to healthful, but we think you'll be pleased with the results.

Most of these sauces were designed to be served with recipes that appear in this book. We decided to group them together in this chapter because they're so good that they shouldn't be relegated to just one dish. Be creative in your use of these delicious, versatile sauces.

Basic Vinaigrette
(with Variations)

"To make a good salad is to be a brilliant diplomatist.
The problem is entirely the same in both cases. To know
how much oil one must mix with one's vinegar."
—Oscar Wilde

MAKES 4 SERVINGS (¼ CUP)   PREPARATION TIME: 5 MINUTES

2 tablespoons extra-virgin olive oil
2 tablespoons balsamic vinegar or wine vinegar
¼ teaspoon Low-Sodium Seasoned Salt (page 297) or salt substitute
   Dash freshly ground black pepper

Combine all ingredients in a small bowl and mix well. Serve on salad greens. Keeps for 2 weeks, refrigerated.

PER SERVING: 61 calories; 7 g fat (96.9% calories from fat); trace protein; trace carbohydrate; trace dietary fiber; 0 mg cholesterol; 86 mg sodium.

Notes
Vinaigrette Variations (add to basic recipe):

Herb Vinaigrette: ½ to 1 teaspoon minced parsley, basil, cilantro, or tarragon, etc.
Garlic Vinaigrette: 1 clove garlic, peeled and minced.
Dijon Vinaigrette: 1 teaspoon Dijon mustard.
Caribbean Vinaigrette: 2 tablespoons lime juice (in place of vinegar) and 1 teaspoon minced cilantro.
Asian Vinaigrette: 2 tablespoons lemon juice (in place of vinegar) and 1 teaspoon low-sodium soy sauce.
Flaxseed Oil Vinaigrette: 2 tablespoons flaxseed oil (in place of olive oil).

Avocado Vinaigrette: ¼ to ½ ripe avocado, processed with basic
   ingredients in food processor or blender until smooth.

Pesto Vinaigrette: 1 tablespoon Pesto (page 296).

Olive Vinaigrette: 1 tablespoon Black Olive Tapenade (page 66).

Farm Dressing and Dip

Not exactly ranch dressing, but close.

MAKES 12 SERVINGS (1½ CUPS)   PREPARATION TIME: 5 MINUTES

½ cup low-fat mayonnaise
½ cup nonfat plain yogurt
½ cup low-fat buttermilk
2 tablespoons grated Parmesan cheese
1 tablespoon chopped chives, fresh or freeze-dried
1 tablespoon garlic powder
½ teaspoon dried oregano
½ teaspoon freshly ground black pepper
½ teaspoon Worcestershire sauce
¼ teaspoon seasoned salt
  Pinch dill

Mix all ingredients together and stir until well blended.

Store covered in refrigerator. Keeps for a week.

PER SERVING: 43 calories; 3 g fat (63.8% calories from fat); 3 g protein; 5 g carbohydrate; trace dietary fiber; 5 mg cholesterol; 111 mg sodium.

SERVING IDEA: Serve this with green salads such as BLT Salad (page 116) or as a dip with vegetables or Crispy Chicken Tenders (page 174).

Note
This basic creamy salad dressing can be jazzed up to suit the salad. For taco salad, add ¼ to ½ teaspoon chili powder; for Middle Eastern, 1 clove minced garlic and 2 tablespoons chopped cilantro; for tropical, ½ teaspoon each grated orange and lemon peel; and for Asian, 1 teaspoon soy sauce and ½ teaspoon sesame oil.

Louie Salad Dressing

A distinctive dressing for Shrimp or Crab Louie.

MAKES 6 SERVINGS (¾ CUP)   PREPARATION TIME: 10 MINUTES

½ cup low-fat mayonnaise
2 tablespoons chili sauce or ketchup
1 teaspoon lemon juice
½ teaspoon Worcestershire sauce
1 tablespoon minced green bell pepper
1 tablespoon minced green onions
   Dash freshly ground black pepper
   Dash salt or salt substitute
1 to 2 tablespoons skim milk

Mix all ingredients except milk with a whisk until smooth. Add milk, a little at a time, until you achieve a creamy, yet pourable consistency.

PER SERVING: 56 calories; 5 g fat (84.9% calories from fat); trace protein; 2 g carbohydrate; trace dietary fiber; 7 mg cholesterol; 101 mg sodium. EXCHANGES: 1 fat.

SERVING IDEA: Serve this with Shrimp Louie (page 121) or other green salads.

Cucumber-Dill Sauce

Great with any kind of fish.

MAKES 6 SERVINGS (1½ CUPS)   PREPARATION TIME: 10 MINUTES

1 *cup nonfat plain yogurt*
¾ *cup peeled and chopped cucumber*
1 *teaspoon freshly chopped dill or ½ teaspoon dried dill*
⅛ *teaspoon freshly ground black pepper*
¼ *teaspoon salt*

Mix all ingredients together in a small bowl. Cover and refrigerate until ready to serve. Keeps in the fridge for about a week.

PER SERVING: 22 calories; trace fat (3.2% calories from fat); 2 g protein; 3 g carbohydrate; trace dietary fiber; 1 mg cholesterol; 118 mg sodium.

SERVING IDEA: Cucumber-Dill Sauce will spruce up any kind of fish. Try it with Broiled Fish Fillets (page 204).

Note
Dill is used in herbal medicine to treat heartburn and other digestive problems, including colic in children.

Homemade Mayonnaise

A basic recipe with delightful variations.

MAKES 16 SERVINGS (1 CUP)   PREPARATION TIME: 10 MINUTES

1 *egg*
2 *teaspoons lemon juice*
¼ *teaspoon salt*
1 *teaspoon Dijon mustard*
¼ *cup extra-virgin olive oil*
¾ *cup almond or walnut oil*

Place egg, lemon juice, salt, and mustard in a blender and process for 30 seconds. With the blender running, remove the lid and slowly add the oil, 1 tablespoon at a time, alternating between the two types. (You may not need a full cup of oil.) Process until thick and smooth. Homemade Mayonnaise may be stored in the refrigerator for at least a week.

PER SERVING (1 tablespoon): 124 calories; 14 g fat (98.6% calories from fat); trace protein; trace carbohydrate; trace dietary fiber; 12 mg cholesterol; 39 mg sodium. EXCHANGE: 1½ fat.

Notes

Every once in a while, Homemade Mayonnaise will curdle, due to atmospheric conditions. If this happens, remove it from the blender. Place another egg in the blender, turn the blender on low, and slowly pour curdled mayonnaise back into the blender. Process until smooth. If it is too thick, add a few drops of water and process again.

(continued)

Homemade Mayonnaise (*continued*)

Real mayonnaise, even this version, is high in fat. However, this one is made with healthful oil and has no additives, so it is much better than brands you'll find in your supermarket. Several of our recipes call for low-fat mayonnaise. If you have a problem with it, use this in its place. Be aware that you'll be adding additional fat calories.

There are many variations on mayonnaise. Olive oil has a strong flavor, so we suggest using another high-quality oil of your choice, or a blend of oils, as we did in this recipe. To make herbal mayonnaise, add 1 tablespoon of chives, basil, or cilantro after adding oil. To make an easy version of aioli (French garlic mayonnaise), add 1 clove minced garlic. For green mayonnaise (nice with fish) add 1½ cups lightly blanched, completely dried spinach or parsley.

Mac's Special Sauce

A pretty close knock-off of McDonald's secret sauce.

MAKES 9 SERVINGS (¾ CUP)   PREPARATION TIME: 10 MINUTES

½ *cup low-fat mayonnaise*
4 *teaspoons sweet pickle relish*
2 *tablespoons ketchup or French salad dressing*
1 *teaspoon vinegar*
1 *tablespoon finely minced onion*
1 *teaspoon xylitol*

In a small bowl, combine all ingredients and stir until well blended. Cover and refrigerate. This will keep in the fridge for a couple of weeks.

PER SERVING: 43 calories; 4 g fat (71.8% calories from fat); trace protein; 3 g carbohydrate; trace dietary fiber; 4 mg cholesterol; 121 mg sodium. EXCHANGE: ½ fat.

SERVING IDEA: This is good on burgers and other sandwiches. Try it on Grilled Turkey Sandwiches (page 102). You may also thin it with a little milk and use it as a salad dressing.

Artichoke Salsa

A tasty topper for fish or chicken.

MAKES 8 SERVINGS (2 CUPS)   PREPARATION TIME: 40 MINUTES

7   *ounces marinated whole artichoke hearts*
½   *cup sliced ripe olives*
¼   *cup chopped onion*
2   *tomatoes, chopped*
3   *cloves garlic, peeled and minced*
2   *tablespoons chopped basil*
¼   *teaspoon Low-Sodium Seasoned Salt (page 297) or salt substitute*
¼   *teaspoon freshly ground black pepper*
⅛   *teaspoon red pepper flakes*

Drain artichoke hearts and coarsely chop. Combine with remaining ingredients in a medium bowl and toss until well blended. Cover and refrigerate at least 30 minutes before serving. This keeps well in the fridge for 4 or 5 days.

PER SERVING: 45 calories; 2 g fat (44.0% calories from fat); 2 g protein; 5 g carbohydrate; 2 g dietary fiber; 0 mg cholesterol; 157 mg sodium. EXCHANGES: 1 vegetable; ½ fat.

SERVING IDEAS: Spoon this over broiled or grilled chicken or fish for a quick and easy entrée. (See recipe for Halibut with Artichoke Salsa on page 210.) It also makes a nice dip with whole wheat pita triangles.

Note
Artichokes contain a substance called cynarine, which makes other things you eat with them taste a little sweeter.

Mary's Fresh Salsa

This recipe is from Mary Fonseca, the incredible cook who organizes all the potlucks and celebrations at the Whitaker Wellness Institute.

MAKES 8 SERVINGS (2 CUPS)   PREPARATION TIME: 20 MINUTES

1   *pound (3 medium) fresh tomatoes, chopped*
1   *small onion, chopped*
½   *cup freshly chopped cilantro*
1   *to 2 small jalapeño chiles (preferably fresh), seeds removed (to taste—they're very hot) and chopped*
3   *cloves garlic, peeled and minced*
½   *teaspoon dried oregano*
½   *teaspoon salt or salt substitute*

Combine all ingredients, adding more or fewer jalapeños to taste. (Handle fresh jalapeños with care.) Do not use a blender or food processor for fresh salsa—it turns out too mushy. This will keep for several days, but gets a little soggy after a day or two.

PER SERVING: 20 calories; trace fat (9.3% calories from fat); 1 g protein; 4 g carbohydrate; 1 g dietary fiber; 0 mg cholesterol; 139 mg sodium. EXCHANGE: 1 vegetable.

SERVING IDEA: Serve this with many Mexican dishes, such as Chicken Fajitas (page 181), Chicken-Chile Quesadillas (page 108), and Mexican Pizza (page 249).

Note

Cilantro doesn't keep very long in a plastic bag in the refrigerator. It lasts much longer if you put it in a sturdy cup or mug half filled with water. Place the stems in the water, like flowers in a vase, and loosely cover the leaves with a plastic bag.

Quick and Easy Salsa
Keeps in the fridge for a week.

MAKES 8 SERVINGS (1½ CUPS)   PREPARATION TIME: 10 MINUTES

1 (14½-ounce) can low-sodium tomatoes with juice, drained and chopped
1 small (4-ounce) can diced green chiles, drained
½ small onion, chopped
1 to 2 small jalapeño chiles (fresh or canned), seeds removed (to taste—they're very hot)
2 cloves garlic, peeled and minced
½ teaspoon dried oregano
½ teaspoon salt or salt substitute

Place all ingredients in a medium bowl and mix well. You may also process in a blender or food processor for 2 to 3 seconds. Do not overprocess or it will be too smooth. This keeps in the refrigerator for at least a week.

PER SERVING: 20 calories; trace fat (4.7% calories from fat); 1 g protein; 4 g carbohydrate; 1 g dietary fiber; 0 mg cholesterol; 158 mg sodium. EXCHANGE: 1 vegetable.

SERVING IDEAS: Serve this with Chicken-Chile Quesadillas (page 108), Chicken Fajitas (page 181), Mexican Pizza (page 249), and other Mexican dishes. You can also marinate chicken breasts or fish fillets in this salsa for an hour, then grill, broil, or bake them.

Note
You can make this as hot or as mild as you please by adjusting the amount of jalapeños. (Including the seeds makes it much hotter.) Handle chile peppers with care—the oils can burn! If you handle a lot of chile peppers, wear disposable latex (surgical) gloves.

Tangy Tartar Sauce
Liven up fish with this tangy sauce.

MAKES 8 SERVINGS (1 CUP)   PREPARATION TIME: 10 MINUTES

½ cup low-fat mayonnaise
¼ cup chopped green onion
¼ cup chopped dill pickle
2 tablespoons lemon juice
¼ teaspoon freshly ground black pepper

Combine all ingredients in a small bowl and mix well. Cover and refrigerate until ready to serve. This sauce keeps well in the refrigerator for a couple of weeks.

PER SERVING: 43 calories; 4 g fat (83.0% calories from fat); trace protein; 2 g carbohydrate; trace dietary fiber; 5 mg cholesterol; 133 mg sodium. EXCHANGE: 1 fat.

SERVING IDEAS: Tangy Tartar Sauce is especially good with Gourmet Fish Sticks (page 203) and Spicy Salmon Cakes (page 200).

Note
Add 1 small can of water-packed tuna, well drained, and voilà! You have quick and healthy tuna salad.

Raita

Cool cucumber sauce from India.

MAKES 10 SERVINGS (3½ CUPS)   PREPARATION TIME: 10 MINUTES

2   *cups nonfat plain yogurt*
1   *medium cucumber, peeled and chopped*
2   *tablespoons freshly chopped cilantro or mint, plus more for
    garnish*
½ *teaspoon ground cumin
    Dash cayenne pepper*

Combine all ingredients in a medium bowl and stir until blended.
Garnish with extra cilantro.

PER SERVING: 31 calories; trace fat (4.6% calories from fat); 3 g protein; 5 g carbohydrate; trace dietary fiber; 1 mg cholesterol; 36 mg
sodium. EXCHANGE: ½ nonfat milk.

SERVING IDEA: Raita is the perfect foil for spicy dishes, particularly
curries and other Indian dishes.

Note

Make sure the yogurt you eat is labeled as having "live and active
cultures." These probiotic bacteria enhance the health of the gas-
trointestinal tract and are being studied for their ability to boost
immune function.

Garlic Sauce

Garlic lovers, this sauce is for you.

<u>MAKES 4 SERVINGS (1 CUP)</u>   PREPARATION TIME: 1 HOUR

1 *cup nonfat plain yogurt*
1 *clove garlic, peeled and minced, or more to taste*
¼ *teaspoon salt or salt substitute*

Place all ingredients in a small bowl and stir to mix well. Let sit in the refrigerator at least an hour before serving. Keeps in a covered container in the refrigerator for 7 to 10 days.

PER SERVING: 35 calories; trace fat (2.8% calories from fat); 3 g protein; 5 g carbohydrate; trace dietary fiber; 1 mg cholesterol; 310 mg sodium. EXCHANGE: ½ nonfat milk.

SERVING IDEAS: Garlic Sauce is a natural with Falafel Sandwiches (page 106), and if you like garlic, it's wonderful for perking up grilled chicken or fish.

Note
The inspiration for this comes from our favorite Middle Eastern restaurant. Don't plan any hot dates after eating this sauce—it's very garlicky.

Lemon-Chive Sauce

Livens up steamed vegetables.

MAKES 4 SERVINGS (½ CUP)   PREPARATION TIME: 10 MINUTES

½ cup low-sodium chicken broth
2 tablespoons lemon juice
2 teaspoons cornstarch
½ teaspoon low-sodium soy sauce
1 teaspoon chopped chives, fresh or freeze-dried
¼ teaspoon xylitol
1 teaspoon butter (preferably organic)

Combine all ingredients except for butter in a small saucepan. Stir until cornstarch is completely dissolved. Slowly bring to a boil over medium heat, stirring constantly. Lower heat and continue cooking and stirring until sauce is thick and bubbly, 3 to 5 minutes.

Remove from heat, add butter, and stir until melted.

Store covered in the refrigerator for 5 to 6 days.

PER SERVING: 23 calories; 1 g fat (35.6% calories from fat); 1 g protein; 2 g carbohydrate; trace dietary fiber; 3 mg cholesterol; 100 mg sodium.

SERVING IDEAS: Serve over broccoli (recipe on page 260), cauliflower, zucchini, or any other steamed vegetable. It's also good with fish.

Note
Fresh lemons are best, but keep a bottle of lemon juice on hand for when you run out of lemons.

Healthy Hollandaise Sauce

Not a dead ringer for the real thing, but much healthier.

MAKES 4 SERVINGS (¾ CUP)   PREPARATION TIME: 15 MINUTES

1½ tablespoons cornstarch
 ⅔ cup skim milk
  1 teaspoon butter (preferably organic)
2½ tablespoons lemon juice
 ¼ teaspoon salt or low sodium salt substitute
  1 egg yolk

Stir cornstarch into milk in a medium saucepan and heat over medium-low heat. Using a wire whisk, stir often while cooking until sauce is thick, about 5 minutes.

Add butter and continue to whisk until melted. Dribble in lemon juice and salt, stirring all the while.

Beat egg yolk lightly. Reduce the heat to low and slowly pour in egg. Whisk until smooth.

PER SERVING: 51 calories; 2 g fat (40.2% calories from fat); 2 g protein; 6 g carbohydrate; trace dietary fiber; 56 mg cholesterol; 166 mg sodium. EXCHANGE: ½ fat.

SERVING IDEAS: This is the best part of the Artichokes with Healthy Hollandaise Sauce (page 261). It also makes a good sauce for chicken, fish, and steamed vegetables.

Note
Hollandaise is traditionally made with lots of egg yolks and butter. This recipe has a minimum of both.

Tomato Cream Sauce

A change from the usual tomato sauce—with a hint of vodka.

MAKES 3 SERVINGS (1 CUP)   PREPARATION TIME: 25 MINUTES

1 teaspoon extra-virgin olive oil
1 small onion, finely chopped
2 cloves garlic, peeled and chopped
1 (14½-ounce) can low-sodium tomatoes with juice, finely chopped
½ cup evaporated milk
2 tablespoons vodka (optional)
¼ teaspoon salt
⅛ teaspoon red pepper flakes
⅛ teaspoon freshly ground black pepper

Heat olive oil in a medium saucepan over medium heat. Add onion and garlic and sauté for 3 or 4 minutes until onion is tender.

Add tomatoes to saucepan and bring to a boil over medium-high heat. Reduce heat and simmer uncovered for 15 minutes until almost dry.

Add evaporated milk, vodka, salt, red pepper flakes and black pepper to saucepan and stir until it begins to boil and sauce thickens.

PER SERVING: 86 calories; 4 g fat (44.4% calories from fat); 3 g protein; 7 g carbohydrate; 1 g dietary fiber; 9 mg cholesterol; 171 mg sodium. EXCHANGES: ½ vegetable; ½ fat.

SERVING IDEAS: Serve this on pasta, steamed vegetables, or chicken.

Mandarin Dipping Sauce
Redolent of soy, ginger, and garlic.

MAKES 8 SERVINGS (½ CUP)   PREPARATION TIME: 10 MINUTES

3 tablespoons low-sodium soy sauce
½ cup water
2 tablespoons rice wine or dry sherry
1 teaspoon grated gingerroot or ½ teaspoon ground ginger
1 clove garlic, peeled and minced

Combine all ingredients in a small saucepan. Bring to a boil over medium-high heat and boil for 1 minute. (Or cook in a microwave for 3 minutes.) Transfer to a covered container and refrigerate. This will keep for a couple of weeks.

PER SERVING: 19 calories; trace fat (1.3% calories from fat); 1 g protein; 1 g carbohydrate; trace dietary fiber; 0 mg cholesterol; 226 mg sodium. EXCHANGE: ½ vegetable.

SERVING IDEA: Serve this with Moo Shoo Vegetables in Lettuce Leaves (page 241), Chicken Satay (page 74), or Grilled Shrimp Brochettes (page 213).

Note
Ginger has been extensively studied for its ability to prevent nausea. To prevent motion sickness, eat 1 to 2 slices of fresh or candied ginger, drink a cup of ginger tea, or take 2 to 4 capsules of powdered ginger just before traveling. For morning sickness during pregnancy, take as needed.

Thai Peanut Sauce

Thai cuisine does wonderful things with peanut butter,
as this recipe attests.

MAKES 6 SERVINGS (¾ CUP)   PREPARATION TIME: 10 MINUTES

½ *cup water*
⅓ *cup peanut butter (natural, without hydrogenated oils)*
1 *tablespoon xylitol*
1 *clove garlic, peeled and chopped*
1 *tablespoon lemon juice*
2 *teaspoons low-sodium soy sauce*
¼ *tablespoon crushed red pepper flakes, or to taste*

Mix all ingredients in a small saucepan and bring to a boil over medium heat. Reduce heat and simmer, stirring often, for 3 to 4 minutes, until sauce is thick and creamy. Transfer to a small serving dish. Serve at room temperature. Keeps in the refrigerator for more than a week.

PER SERVING: 92 calories; 7 g fat (64.4% calories from fat); 4 g protein; 5 g carbohydrate; 1 g dietary fiber; 0 mg cholesterol; 134 mg sodium. EXCHANGES: ½ lean meat; 1 fat.

SERVING IDEAS: Serve this as a dipping sauce with Chicken Satay (page 74) or Grilled Shrimp Brochettes (page 213). This sauce can also be thinned with a teaspoon of olive oil and a little water and used as a dressing on an Asian-style salad.

Note

The reason most commercial brands of peanut butter are so smooth and creamy is because they have been hydrogenated, or processed to make their liquid oils solid at room temperature. Trans fatty acids are a by-product of this process, and excessive consumption of trans fats increases risk of heart disease.

Gravy

A basic gravy recipe with a minimum of fat and fuss.

MAKES 8 SERVINGS (2 CUPS)   PREPARATION TIME: 15 MINUTES

2 *tablespoons hazelnut oil or olive oil or drippings (see Notes)*
3 *tablespoons unbleached flour*
2 *cups low-sodium chicken broth*
⅛ *teaspoon freshly ground black pepper*

Heat hazelnut oil over medium heat. Add flour and cook, stirring constantly, for 1 to 2 minutes.

Slowly pour in chicken broth while stirring with a whisk. Bring to a boil, reduce heat, and simmer, stirring often until thickened. Season with pepper.

PER SERVING: 52 calories; 3 g fat (57.8% calories from fat); 3 g protein; 3 g carbohydrate; trace dietary fiber; 0 mg cholesterol; 130 mg sodium. EXCHANGES: ½ lean meat; ½ fat.

SERVING IDEAS: Serve this with Pecan Stuffing (page 269) and Two-Hour Roasted Turkey (page 187), or spruce up any grain with a spoonful of Gravy.

Notes

If you want thicker gravy, stir 1 tablespoon cornstarch into 2 tablespoons cold water, add to gravy, and stir until desired thickness is achieved. If you want thinner gravy, add more chicken broth, 1 to 2 tablespoons at a time.

If you have drippings from a roasted turkey or chicken, use in place of hazelnut or olive oil. Scrape the drippings into a medium saucepan, omit the oil, add the flour, then proceed with the recipe.

Homemade Marinara Sauce

A healthy, easy version of spaghetti sauce.

MAKES 8 SERVINGS (4 CUPS)   PREPARATION TIME: 45 MINUTES

1   large (28-ounce) can low-sodium tomatoes with juice, chopped,
    juice reserved
¼   cup tomato paste
1   medium onion, chopped
1   green bell pepper, seeded and chopped
3   cloves garlic, peeled and minced
1   teaspoon oregano
2   tablespoons freshly chopped basil leaves or 1 teaspoon dried
    basil
½   teaspoon salt or salt substitute
¼   teaspoon freshly ground black pepper

Combine all ingredients in a medium saucepan. Bring to a boil over medium-high heat, then reduce heat and simmer, uncovered, stirring occasionally, for 30 minutes.

PER SERVING: 37 calories; trace fat (5.1% calories from fat); 2 g protein; 9 g carbohydrate; 2 g dietary fiber; 0 mg cholesterol; 211 mg sodium. EXCHANGE: 1½ vegetable.

SERVING IDEA: Serve this on pasta or use in recipes calling for spaghetti sauce, such as Lasagna Roll-Ups (page 223).

Note

This can be halved for a single recipe or doubled and stored in a covered container in the refrigerator for 5 to 6 days. It's an excellent substitute for canned spaghetti sauce, which usually contains lots of sodium.

Fresh Cranberry-Orange Relish

*No cooking required—and much better
than canned cranberry sauce.*

MAKES 10 SERVINGS (2½ CUPS)   PREPARATION TIME: 10 MINUTES

12 *ounces fresh or frozen cranberries*
 1 *tablespoon grated orange peel*
 1 *medium orange, peeled and seeded*
 ¾ *cup xylitol, or to taste*

Place cranberries, orange peel, and orange in a food processor or blender and process, turning on and off, until evenly chopped. Do not overprocess.

Transfer to a medium bowl and add xylitol, beginning with ½ cup and adding more until desired sweetness is achieved. (Don't overdo it—this should be tart.) This will keep in the refrigerator 7 to 10 days.

PER SERVING: 58 calories; trace fat (0.9% calories from fat); trace protein; 20 g carbohydrate; 2 g dietary fiber; 0 mg cholesterol; trace sodium. EXCHANGE: ½ fruit.

SERVING IDEA: Serve with Two-Hour Roasted Turkey (page 187). It makes a nice relish with any poultry or meat.

Note

Compounds in cranberry called proanthocyanidins prevent bacteria from sticking to the urinary tract walls and causing infection. They also protect the stomach lining from invasion by *H. pylori* bacteria, helping guard against ulcers.

Pesto

An explosion of flavor—dresses up any fish,
poultry, or vegetable dish.

MAKES 6 SERVINGS (½ CUP)   PREPARATION TIME: 10 MINUTES

1   *tablespoon pine nuts (optional)*
1   *clove garlic, peeled*
1   *cup fresh basil leaves, tightly packed*
¼   *cup grated Parmesan cheese*
¼   *cup fresh parsley, tightly packed*
3   *tablespoons extra-virgin olive oil*

In a food processor or blender, process pine nuts, garlic, basil, Parmesan, and parsley until chopped. Slowly add olive oil through the opening on top of the food processor while running, and continue to process until smooth. Scrape the sides occasionally to make sure pesto is well blended. Pesto keeps refrigerated in a covered container for at least a week.

PER SERVING: 86 calories; 9 g fat (88.5% calories from fat); 2 g protein; 1 g carbohydrate; trace dietary fiber; 3 mg cholesterol; 65 mg sodium. EXCHANGE: 1½ fat.

SERVING IDEAS: Pesto is extremely versatile. Use it in Grilled Pesto Vegetables (page 253), brush it on fish or poultry, or stir it into pasta. It also makes a wonderful sandwich spread and a zesty addition to vinaigrette salad dressing. Yes, it's high in fat, but it's good fat—and a little bit goes a long way.

Low-Sodium Seasoned Salt
A reduced-sodium seasoning.

MAKES ¾ CUP   PREPARATION TIME: 10 MINUTES

3 tablespoons salt or salt substitute
1 tablespoon onion powder
1 tablespoon garlic powder
1 tablespoon chili powder
1 teaspoon ground cumin
1 teaspoon dried marjoram
1 teaspoon paprika
½ teaspoon curry powder

Combine all ingredients in a jar with a tight-fitting lid. Shake well until thoroughly blended.

PER SERVING (⅛ teaspoon): trace calories; trace fat; trace protein; trace carbohydrate; trace dietary fiber; 0 mg cholesterol; 67 mg sodium.

Note
This is a low-sodium alternative to regular salt. If you are salt-sensitive, use a salt substitute, such as Nu-Salt, which contains potassium chloride and no sodium at all. You may add as much Nu-Salt to this as you want.

No-Salt Herbal Seasoning

Bursting with flavor—and just a trace of sodium.

MAKES ¼ CUP   PREPARATION TIME: 10 MINUTES

1 *tablespoon dried parsley*
1 *tablespoon onion powder*
1 *tablespoon garlic powder*
1 *teaspoon freshly ground black pepper*
1 *teaspoon dried basil*
1 *teaspoon dried thyme*
1 *teaspoon dried marjoram*
½ *teaspoon dried oregano*

Mix all ingredients together in a small lidded jar or covered bowl. Stir or shake until well blended. Store covered.

PER SERVING (⅛ teaspoon): 1 calorie; trace fat; trace protein; trace carbohydrate; trace dietary fiber; 0 mg cholesterol; trace sodium.

SERVING IDEA: Spice up any dish with this herbal blend, or use in place of Mrs. Dash or other salt-free seasonings.

Desserts

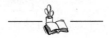

Just because you have diabetes doesn't mean you have to banish dessert from your life. You do need to be more selective in your choices, because popular desserts such as cakes, brownies, pies, and cookies contain lots of hydrogenated and saturated fat as well as flour, sugar, and other refined carbohydrates that drive up blood sugar. Don't despair, for you are still left with a multitude of sweet selections. These include fresh fruit desserts such as Granny's Apples (page 302) and Peaches 'n' Devonshire Cream (page 300), baked Blueberry Crumble (page 314) and Apple-Pear Crisp (page 313), and gourmet Cherry Crepes (page 316) and Chocolate-Dipped Strawberries (page 308).

A rule of thumb for enjoying dessert is moderation. The purpose of dessert is to cap off a meal or satisfy an occasional sweet tooth, so keep serving sizes small.

Peaches 'n' Devonshire Cream

Equally good with fresh or frozen peaches.

MAKES 4 SERVINGS   PREPARATION TIME: 20 MINUTES

3 cups peeled and sliced peaches (fresh or frozen, defrosted)
1 tablespoon plus 1 teaspoon xylitol
½ cup low-fat sour cream
1 teaspoon honey
¼ teaspoon vanilla extract

Place peaches and 1 tablespoon xylitol in a medium bowl and toss to coat well. (Xylitol is optional.) Cover and refrigerate for 10 minutes.

Meanwhile, make Devonshire Cream by combining sour cream, 1 teaspoon xylitol, honey, and vanilla in a small bowl and mixing well.

Divide peaches among four dessert dishes and top each with a dollop of Devonshire Cream.

PER SERVING: 106 calories; 2 g fat (11.7% calories from fat); 3 g protein; 23 g carbohydrate; 3 g dietary fiber; 9 mg cholesterol; 34 mg sodium. EXCHANGES: 1 fruit; ½ fat; ½ other carbohydrates.

SERVING IDEAS: Devonshire Cream is always a big hit. It's also delicious with fresh berries.

Note

Fresh peaches are pretty iffy most of the year. Frozen sliced peaches, which come in big bags so you can take out as many as you need and reseal, are surprisingly good. Do not purchase peaches packed in syrup.

Razzle-Dazzle Raspberries
An easy way to gussy up fresh berries.

MAKES 4 SERVINGS   PREPARATION TIME: 10 MINUTES

2 *tablespoons Grand Marnier or other liqueur*
½ *teaspoon shredded orange peel*
2 *cups fresh raspberries*
8 *tablespoons pressurized whipped cream (preferably light)*

Combine Grand Marnier and orange peel in a medium bowl. Add raspberries and lightly stir to coat.

Divide raspberries among four dessert dishes. Top each with 2 tablespoons whipped cream.

PER SERVING: 78 calories; 2 g fat (27.5% calories from fat); 1 g protein; 11 g carbohydrate; 4 g dietary fiber; 6 mg cholesterol; 10 mg sodium. EXCHANGES: ½ fruit; ½ fat.

SERVING IDEA: Blueberries, blackberries, or other fresh berries can be substituted.

Note
Of all fruits and vegetables, berries contain the most antioxidants, with blueberries leading the pack.

Granny's Apples

A light, easy, and healthy ending to a meal.

MAKES 4 SERVINGS   PREPARATION TIME: 10 MINUTES

2 *large Granny Smith apples*
4 *tablespoons frozen apple juice concentrate*
2 *tablespoons lemon juice*
4 *drops stevia, or to taste*
  Dash ground cinnamon

Scrub and core apples (do not peel) and cut into very, very thin slices. Place in a medium serving bowl.

Mix apple juice concentrate, lemon juice, stevia, and cinnamon in a small bowl.

Pour apple juice mixture over apples and toss to coat. Serve at once or refrigerate.

PER SERVING: 62 calories; trace fat (1.8% calories from fat); trace protein; 16 g carbohydrate; 1 g dietary fiber; 0 mg cholesterol; 6 mg sodium. EXCHANGE: 1 fruit.

Note

These apples are even better after they've marinated in the refrigerator for a few hours. The lemon juice prevents the apple slices from turning brown.

Mini Grape-Sicles

Kids especially like these frozen grape "Popsicles."

MAKES 4 SERVINGS   PREPARATION TIME: 1 HOUR 10 MINUTES

¾ *pound (1 medium bunch) seedless grapes*
   Wooden toothpicks

Pick grapes off stems. Place 3 grapes on each toothpick, leaving enough toothpick exposed on one end to pick it up.

Place on a plate or baking sheet and freeze until hard, about an hour. Eat them right away or store in a sealed plastic bag in the freezer.

PER SERVING: 34 calories; trace fat (2.2% calories from fat); trace protein; 9 g carbohydrate; 1 g dietary fiber; 0 mg cholesterol; 5 mg sodium. EXCHANGE: ½ fruit.

SERVING IDEA: You can also freeze grapes without the toothpicks and serve in parfait glasses or wineglasses.

Note

Growing grapes, which are technically berries, is the world's biggest single food industry. Grape skins and particularly grape seeds are an abundant source of compounds called oligomeric proanthocyanidins (OPCs), which have more antioxidant power than vitamin C, vitamin E, and beta-carotene. OPCs have also been shown to help strengthen the blood vessels and protect against cardiovascular disease.

Poached Pears with
Rich Chocolate Sauce

An elegant way to serve fruit—and the chocolate sauce is to die for.

MAKES 4 SERVINGS   PREPARATION TIME: 1 HOUR

2 *cups water*
½ *cup xylitol*
1 *teaspoon vanilla extract*
2 *large ripe, firm pears, peeled, halved, and cored*
4 *tablespoons Bret's Rich Chocolate Sauce (page 305)*

In a large saucepan, combine water, xylitol, and vanilla, and bring to a boil.

Add pears, reduce heat, and simmer for 15 minutes, basting with water occasionally. Remove from the heat and let pears cool in sugar water for 15 minutes.

Remove pears and refrigerate until chilled, at least 45 minutes.

Place pears in four bowls and spoon 1 tablespoon Bret's Rich Chocolate Sauce over each.

PER SERVING (including Rich Chocolate Sauce): 149 calories; 2 g fat (10.6% calories from fat); 1 g protein; 43 g carbohydrate; 3 g dietary fiber; 0 mg cholesterol; 6 mg sodium. EXCHANGES: 1 fruit; ½ fat; ½ other carbohydrates.

Note
All firm fruits such as pears, apples, nectarines, and peaches take well to poaching. Simply cover whole or coarsely chopped fruit with water, sweetened with a natural sweetener and flavored with vanilla or almond extract, cinnamon, cloves, or nutmeg. Poached fruit is good as a dessert or a topping on cereal or yogurt.

Bret's Rich Chocolate Sauce
*This one's named for a guy who gives new meaning
to the term* chocoholic.

MAKES 8 SERVINGS (½ CUP)   PREPARATION TIME: 20 MINUTES

1 *cup plus 1 teaspoon water*
⅓ *cup semisweet chocolate chips*
1 *tablespoon xylitol*
1 *teaspoon cornstarch*
½ *teaspoon vanilla extract*

Place cup of water, chocolate chips, and xylitol in a small saucepan and bring to a boil over medium heat. Reduce heat and simmer for 15 minutes.

Meanwhile, stir cornstarch into teaspoon of water. Pour cornstarch mixture into saucepan, stirring constantly until thickened. Remove from heat and stir in vanilla. It keeps for about a week in the refrigerator. Reheat before serving.

PER SERVING (sauce only): 39 calories; 2 g fat (41.7% calories from fat); 1 g protein; 6 g carbohydrate; 1 g dietary fiber; trace cholesterol; 2 mg sodium. EXCHANGES: 1 fat; ½ other carbohydrates.

SERVING IDEA: Serve over poached pears or other desserts. A little bit goes a long way.

Note
Cocoa and dark chocolate are concentrated sources of the same antioxidant-rich flavenoids that give green tea and red wine their health benefits.

Dessert Fondue

Fondue has made a comeback. This is a healthy version.

MAKES 4 SERVINGS   PREPARATION TIME: 20 MINUTES

⅓ cup frozen apple juice concentrate
2 tablespoons brown rice syrup
1 teaspoon lemon juice
½ teaspoon ground cinnamon
   Dash ground cloves
1 tablespoon cornstarch
⅓ cup water
1 tablespoon butter (preferably organic)
1 large apple, cored and sliced
1 large pear, cored and sliced

Place apple juice concentrate, brown rice syrup, lemon juice, cinnamon, and cloves in a small saucepan. Heat over medium heat, stirring often, until boiling, about 3 minutes. Reduce the heat to a simmer.

Meanwhile, stir cornstarch into water and add to saucepan. Stir constantly as mixture thickens for 2 minutes. Turn off heat; stir in butter until melted.

Transfer to a small serving bowl. Arrange apple and pear slices around the bowl. Dip fruit into the warm fondue.

PER SERVING: 159 calories; 3 g fat (17.1% calories from fat); 1 g protein; 35 g carbohydrate; 2 g dietary fiber; 8 mg cholesterol; 47 mg sodium. EXCHANGES: 1½ fruit; ½ fat.

SERVING IDEA: Strawberries, banana slices, and other fruit may also be served with Dessert Fondue.

Dessert Pizza

Kids especially like the idea of eating pizza for dessert.

MAKES 8 SLICES   PREPARATION TIME: 20 MINUTES

½ cup softened low-fat cream cheese
4 teaspoons xylitol
¼ teaspoon ground cinnamon
2 medium whole wheat tortillas
½ teaspoon hazelnut oil or almond oil
1 cup blueberries
1 cup strawberries

Preheat the broiler.

Mix cream cheese and 2 teaspoons xylitol in a small bowl and stir until blended.

Mix cinnamon and 2 teaspoons xylitol in a small bowl. Brush tortillas with hazelnut oil and sprinkle with cinnamon-xylitol mixture.

Place tortillas under the broiler, 5 to 6 inches from the heat source, for 2 to 3 minutes, until lightly browned. Cool slightly.

Spread cheese on tortillas and arrange berries on top. Cut each tortilla into quarters and serve.

PER SERVING: 148 calories; 6 g fat (32.2% calories from fat); 5 g protein; 24 g carbohydrate; 2 g dietary fiber; 16 mg cholesterol; 286 mg sodium. EXCHANGES: 1 grain (starch); ½ lean meat; ½ fruit.

Note
A great thing about fruit desserts is that they're so versatile. Try this with orange or kiwi slices, banana (make sure it's barely ripe), or other berries.

Chocolate-Dipped Strawberries

Our most decadent recipe—save it for special occasions.

MAKES 16 TO 24 STRAWBERRIES   PREPARATION TIME: 1 HOUR 15 MINUTES

1 *pound large strawberries, stems intact*
6 *ounces (1 cup) semisweet chocolate chips*

Line a large cookie sheet (but small enough to fit in your refrigerator) with waxed paper.

Rinse strawberries and dry completely. (As little as a drop or two of water can make melted chocolate turn grainy.)

Put chocolate chips in a microwave-proof bowl or glass measuring cup. Microwave for 1 minute, stir, and check chocolate—it should be smooth and glossy. If it isn't, cook another minute, then stir and check again. Continue cooking and checking at 30-second intervals until chocolate is thin enough to dip. (You may also use a double boiler to melt chocolate.)

Holding each strawberry by its stem, dip about halfway into chocolate. Place on waxed paper. If chocolate gets too thick, put back in the microwave for 15 to 20 seconds.

Place cookie sheet in the fridge and let strawberries cool for at least an hour, until the chocolate is hard.

PER SERVING (2 or 3 strawberries, depending on size): 118 calories; 7 g fat (44.5% calories from fat); 1 g protein; 17 g carbohydrate; 2 g dietary fiber; 0 mg cholesterol; 3 mg sodium. EXCHANGES: ½ fruit; 1½ fat; 1 other carbohydrates.

Note
Purchase organic strawberries, if available. Strawberry cultivation involves the use of more pesticides per acre than any other crop.

Fresh Orange Sorbet

Sweet, tart, refreshing—and loaded with vitamin C.

MAKES 4 SERVINGS   PREPARATION TIME: 4 HOURS

4 *cups orange juice (preferably freshly squeezed)*
2 *tablespoons Grand Marnier or Cointreau (optional)*
¼ *teaspoon orange extract*

Mix all ingredients and pour into ice cube trays or a large shallow baking dish. Freeze until firm, several hours or overnight.

Remove from the freezer. Pop frozen juice out of ice cube trays or break into pieces in the baking dish with a heavy spoon.

Place into a food processor or blender and process until smooth. Serve immediately.

PER SERVING: 139 calories; trace fat (3.5% calories from fat); 2 g protein; 29 g carbohydrate; trace dietary fiber; 0 mg cholesterol; 2 mg sodium. EXCHANGE: 2 fruit.

SERVING IDEA: Leftover sorbet will keep in the freezer for a few days. Before serving, process again in a food processor or blender.

Note
Sorbet, which is French for "sherbet," is a smooth, frozen delicacy consisting primarily of fruit juice or puree, water, and a sweetener. If you want this to be sweeter, add a little xylitol.

Crispy Cookie Bars

Sweet enough to satisfy the most avid sweet tooth.

MAKES 16 BARS   PREPARATION TIME: 45 MINUTES

2   *cups old-fashioned rolled oats*
1   *cup raw sunflower seeds*
½   *cup oat bran*
½   *cup brown rice syrup*
⅓   *cup whole wheat flour*
1   *tablespoon hazelnut oil or almond oil*
2   *teaspoons vanilla extract*
    Cooking oil spray (see Note)

Preheat the oven to 300 degrees F.

Spread rolled oats, sunflower seeds, and oat bran evenly over a large shallow 9-by-13-inch baking dish. Bake for 20 minutes, stirring once.

Meanwhile, combine brown rice syrup, flour, and oil in a small saucepan over medium heat. Cook until hot, but not quite boiling, 2 to 3 minutes. Remove from heat and stir in vanilla.

Increase the oven temperature to 350 degrees F. Spray a cookie sheet with oil.

Transfer oats mixture to a large mixing bowl. Pour syrup mixture over oats and stir well to coat evenly.

Using your hands, press onto prepared cookie sheet. (It will be sticky. To make it easier and less messy, put your hand in a plastic bag, and spray a little cooking oil on the bag, and press.) Bars will be thin.

Bake for 10 minutes. Remove from the oven, cool for 10 minutes, then cut into 16 bars. (If you cool longer than this, you won't be able to cut into neat bars.)

PER SERVING (1 bar): 156 calories; 6 g fat (32.6% calories from fat); 5 g protein; 24 g carbohydrate; 3 g dietary fiber; 0 mg cholesterol; 12 mg sodium. EXCHANGES: 1 grain (starch); 1 fat.

Note
Because of its strong flavor, olive oil spray isn't ideal for desserts. Rather than using inferior-quality cooking oil sprays, purchase an oil mister and fill it with almond or hazelnut oil.

Coconut Macaroons

And you thought coconut was off limits . . .

MAKES 18 MACAROONS   PREPARATION TIME: 40 MINUTES

Cooking oil spray
2 egg whites
1⅓ cups shredded coconut
⅓ cup xylitol
3 tablespoons unbleached flour
Dash salt
½ teaspoon almond extract

Preheat the oven to 325 degrees F. Spray a cookie sheet with cooking oil.

Beat egg whites with a wire whisk in a small bowl.

In a large mixing bowl, combine coconut, xylitol, flour, and salt. Stir in egg whites and almond extract and mix well.

Drop 18 teaspoonfuls of coconut mixture onto the prepared cookie sheet. Bake for 20 to 25 minutes, until edges of cookies are golden brown.

Remove from the cookie sheet and cool on a wire rack.

PER SERVING (2 macaroons): 72 calories; 4 g fat (42.3% calories from fat); 2 g protein; 11 g carbohydrate; 1 g dietary fiber; 0 mg cholesterol; 44 mg sodium. EXCHANGE: 1 fat.

Note
Coconut has a bad, and undeserved, reputation because of its high level of saturated fat. However, the fatty acids in coconut oil are easily burned for energy, so they're less apt to contribute to weight gain. Furthermore, half of the fatty acids in coconut oil are lauric acid, which has antiviral and antibacterial properties.

Apple-Pear Crisp

A delectable dessert that can be made with
any combination of fresh fruits.

MAKES 9 SERVINGS   PREPARATION TIME: 1 HOUR 10 MINUTES

  Cooking oil spray
2 medium apples, peeled, cored, and cut into 1-inch pieces
2 medium firm pears, peeled, cored, and cut into 1-inch pieces
¼ cup frozen apple juice concentrate
1 tablespoon lemon juice
1 tablespoon plus ⅓ cup whole wheat flour
1 teaspoon ground cinnamon
1 cup uncooked oatmeal
2 tablespoons hazelnut oil or almond oil
¼ cup chopped walnuts
2 tablespoons brown rice syrup

Preheat the oven to 350 degrees F. Spray an 8-by-8-inch baking dish with cooking oil spray.

Mix apples and pears in a medium mixing bowl. Pour apple juice concentrate, lemon juice, 1 tablespoon flour, and ½ teaspoon cinnamon over fruit. Stir well and pour into the baking dish.

In another mixing bowl, combine ⅓ cup flour, ½ teaspoon cinnamon, oatmeal, hazelnut oil, walnuts, and brown rice syrup and mix well. Sprinkle over fruit in the baking dish.

Bake for 40 to 50 minutes, or until brown and bubbly.

PER SERVING: 173 calories; 6 g fat (29.1% calories from fat); 3 g protein; 29 g carbohydrate; 4 g dietary fiber; 0 mg cholesterol; 8 mg sodium. EXCHANGES: 1 grain (starch); 1 fruit; 1 fat.

Blueberry Crumble

Rich, sweet, and bursting with antioxidants.

MAKES 8 SERVINGS   PREPARATION TIME: 50 MINUTES

4 *cups fresh or frozen blueberries (if frozen, thaw and pat dry)*
¼ *cup tapioca*
4 *tablespoons xylitol*
⅓ *cup whole wheat flour*
3 *tablespoons butter (preferably organic), softened*
2 *tablespoons brown rice syrup*
⅛ *teaspoon ground nutmeg*

Mix blueberries, tapioca, and 2 tablespoons xylitol in a medium bowl. Let sit for 15 minutes.

Preheat the oven to 375 degrees F. Pour blueberries into an 8- or 9-inch pie pan.

In a small bowl, mix flour, butter, remaining xylitol, brown rice syrup, and nutmeg with a fork until coarse crumbs form. Sprinkle over blueberries.

Bake until berries are bubbly and topping is golden brown, 30 to 35 minutes.

PER SERVING: 135 calories; 3 g fat (20.5% calories from fat); 1 g protein; 30 g carbohydrate; 3 g dietary fiber; 8 mg cholesterol; 40 mg sodium. EXCHANGES: ½ grain (starch); ½ fruit; ½ fat.

SERVING IDEA: Serve with a tablespoon of Devonshire Cream (page 300) or light whipped cream, if desired.

French Apple Cake

A nice dessert to serve at a dinner party.

SERVES 8   PREPARATION TIME: 55 MINUTES

4 *(about 2 pounds) Granny Smith apples*
   Cooking oil spray
½ *cup whole wheat flour (preferably pastry)*
⅓ *cup xylitol*
1 *tablespoon baking powder*
   Dash salt
½ *teaspoon vanilla extract*
2 *large eggs, lightly beaten*
2 *tablespoons hazelnut oil or almond oil*
⅓ *cup low-fat 2 percent milk or nonfat milk*

Peel and core apples and cut into thin wedges.

Preheat the oven to 400 degrees F. Spray a 9-inch springform pan with oil.

Combine flour, xylitol, baking powder, and salt in a large bowl. Stir well. Add vanilla, eggs, hazelnut oil, and milk and stir until blended. Add apples and stir until coated with batter.

Pour cake into the prepared pan and bake 20 to 25 minutes, until golden brown and firm to the touch.

Cool on a rack for 10 minutes, then remove the sides of the pan. Cut into eighths.

PER SERVING: 129 calories; 5 g fat (30.3% calories from fat); 3 g protein; 22 g carbohydrate; 2 g dietary fiber; 48 mg cholesterol; 237 mg sodium. EXCHANGES: ½ grain (starch); ½ fruit; 1 fat.

SERVING IDEA: Serve with a dollop of Devonshire Cream (page 300).

Cherry Crepes

Save this show-off dessert for special occasions.

MAKES 8 CREPES   PREPARATION TIME: 45 MINUTES

½ cup unbleached flour
    Pinch salt
¼ cup water
¼ cup skim milk
2 egg whites or ¼ cup Egg Beaters or other egg white product
1 tablespoon xylitol
1 tablespoon hazelnut oil or almond oil
1 tablespoon Grand Marnier or Cointreau (optional)
1 (14-ounce) can cherries with juice
1½ teaspoons cornstarch
    Cooking oil spray

Mix flour and salt in a medium bowl and stir. Mix water and milk and slowly pour into flour mixture, whisking all the while, until smooth. Whisk in egg whites, xylitol, hazelnut oil, and Grand Marnier until completely free of lumps. Let stand in the refrigerator for 45 minutes.

Meanwhile, drain cherries and pour juice into a medium saucepan. Remove 2 tablespoons of juice and mix with cornstarch.

Heat cherry juice over medium heat. Add cornstarch mixture and heat until it begins to boil. Reduce heat and cook for 2 minutes, stirring continuously, until juice thickens. Add cherries and cook, stirring, until cherries are hot. Remove from heat and keep warm.

Heat a small nonstick skillet over medium-high heat until a drop of water dances on the skillet. Spray with oil. Pour ¼ cup of batter into the center of the skillet and quickly swirl the skillet around until batter coats the bottom. Pour out any excess batter. Cook for 30 seconds or until crepe is lightly browned. Jerk the skillet to dislodge crepe, then turn with a spatula or your fingers, or flip it over. Cook on other side for 15 to 20 seconds. Transfer to a wire rack. (Wait until they're cool before stacking them or they'll stick together.)

Spoon cherry mixture onto a strip in the center of each crepe. Fold one side over, then roll from middle toward other side. Serve at once.

PER SERVING: 165 calories; 5 g fat (25% calories from fat); 5 g protein; 26 g carbohydrate; 1 g dietary fiber; 47 mg cholesterol; 71 mg sodium. EXCHANGES: 1 grain (starch); ½ fruit; 1 fat.

SERVING IDEA: Crepes are extremely versatile. They may be filled with any kind of sweetened fruit or sauce—or turned into a main dish by rolling up leftovers of any of the chicken, fish, or vegetarian dishes in this cookbook.

Note

Cherries contain anti-inflammatory phytonutrients that are ten times more powerful than aspirin, and much safer. Just twenty cherries equal the anti-inflammatory effects of one or two aspirin tablets. Those same twenty cherries also provide antioxidant protection comparable to that of vitamin C or E.

Lemon Parfaits

A beautiful dessert served in parfait or wineglasses.

MAKES 4 SERVINGS   PREPARATION TIME: 1 HOUR

2½ *cups plain nonfat yogurt*
15   *drops stevia, to taste*
¾   *cup Tart Lemon Dessert Sauce (page 319)*
4   *slices lemon peel, for garnish*

Measure yogurt into a medium bowl and add stevia, 5 drops at a time, until you achieve desired sweetness.

Place 1 tablespoon of yogurt in the bottom of each of 4 white wine or parfait glasses. Carefully spread 1 tablespoon chilled Tart Lemon Dessert Sauce over yogurt, spreading to edges of glass. Gently layer 4 tablespoons of yogurt on sauce, spreading evenly. Spoon in 2 more tablespoons of sauce, followed by 4 more tablespoons of yogurt.

Peel 2 thin 1-inch slices of lemon rind off a cleaned lemon. Cut into very thin strips and place 3 or 4 on each parfait as a garnish.

PER SERVING (includes Tart Lemon Dessert Sauce): 144 calories; 3 g fat (17.7% calories from fat); 8 g protein; 26 g carbohydrate; 0 g dietary fiber; 11 mg cholesterol; 139 mg sodium. EXCHANGES: 1 nonfat milk; ½ fat.

SERVING IDEA: If you're in a hurry, spoon yogurt into bowls and top with Lemon Dessert Sauce.

Tart Lemon Dessert Sauce
This sweet-tart sauce enhances any dessert.

MAKES 4 SERVINGS (¾ CUP)   PREPARATION TIME: 15 MINUTES

¼ cup xylitol
1 tablespoon cornstarch
⅛ teaspoon ground nutmeg
½ cup boiling water
1 tablespoon butter (preferably organic)
1 tablespoon finely grated lemon peel
3 tablespoons lemon juice (juice of 1 lemon)

Place xylitol, cornstarch, and nutmeg in a small saucepan and stir until well mixed.

Gradually pour in boiling water, stirring constantly, and bring to a boil over medium heat. Reduce heat and simmer, stirring for 2 to 3 minutes. Sauce will be thick.

Remove from heat. Stir in butter, lemon peel, and lemon juice. Store in refrigerator.

PER SERVING (sauce only): 65 calories; 3 g fat (30.3% calories from fat); trace protein; 15 g carbohydrate; trace dietary fiber; 8 mg cholesterol; 30 mg sodium. EXCHANGE: ½ fat.

Note
For an even lower-carbohydrate version, substitute stevia for the xylitol. Add 2 to 3 drops at a time, tasting after each addition.

"Reese's Cup" Mousse

The dynamic duo of chocolate and peanut butter in a creamy mousse.

MAKES 5 SERVINGS   PREPARATION TIME: 1 HOUR 10 MINUTES

⅓ cup peanut butter (natural, without hydrogenated fats)
½ cup xylitol
⅓ cup cocoa powder
12 ounces silken tofu (see Note)
1½ teaspoons vanilla extract
 2 tablespoons skim milk

Combine all ingredients in a food processor or blender and process just until smooth.

Place in individual serving dishes and refrigerate at least an hour before serving.

PER SERVING: 219 calories; 13 g fat (42.7% calories from fat); 11 g protein; 28 g carbohydrate; 4 g dietary fiber; trace cholesterol; 89 mg sodium. EXCHANGES: ½ grain (starch); 1½ lean meat; 2 fat.

SERVING IDEA: Serve this in parfait glasses or wineglasses for a beautiful presentation.

Note

Whereas firm or extra firm tofu is best for main dishes because it holds its shape, silken tofu is softer and has a smooth, creamy, custardlike texture appropriate for puddings, pie fillings, dips, and salad dressings. You'll often find silken tofu in 10- to 12-ounce boxes with the Asian foods in your grocery store, as opposed to the refrigerated section, where you'll find firm tofu.

Measurement Conversions

1 ounce		28.35 grams
8 ounces	½ pound	226.8 grams
16 ounces	1 pound	453.6 grams
32 ounces	2 pounds	910 grams
	2 pounds + 3 ounces	1 kilogram or 1,000 grams
¼ teaspoon		1.23 milliliters
½ teaspoon		2.46 milliliters
¾ teaspoon		3.7 milliliters
1 teaspoon		4.93 milliliters
1¼ teaspoons		6.16 milliliters
1½ teaspoons		7.39 milliliters
1¾ teaspoons		8.63 milliliters
2 teaspoons		9.86 milliliters
1 tablespoon		14.79 milliliters
1 fluid ounce		29.57 milliliters
2 tablespoons		29.57 milliliters
¼ cup		59.15 milliliters
½ cup		118.3 milliliters
1 cup		236.59 milliliters
2 cups	1 pint	473.18 milliliters
3 cups		709.77 milliliters
4 cups	1 quart	946.36 milliliters
4 quarts	1 gallon	3.785 liters

½ teaspoon = 30 drops

1 teaspoon = ⅓ tablespoon

3 teaspoons = 1 tablespoon or ½ fluid ounce

½ tablespoon = 1½ teaspoons

1 tablespoon = 3 teaspoons or ½ fluid ounce

2 tablespoons = 1 fluid ounce

3 tablespoons = 1½ fluid ounces or 1 jigger

4 tablespoons = ¼ cup or 2 fluid ounces

5⅓ tablespoons = ⅓ cup

8 tablespoons = ½ cup or 4 fluid ounces

12 tablespoons = ¾ cup or 6 fluid ounces

16 tablespoons = 1 cup or 8 fluid ounces or ½ pint

⅛ cup = 2 tablespoons or 1 fluid ounce

¼ cup = 4 tablespoons or 2 fluid ounces

⅓ cup = 5 tablespoons + 1 teaspoon

½ cup = 8 tablespoons or 4 fluid ounces or 1 gill

¾ cup = 12 tablespoons or 6 fluid ounces

1 cup = 16 tablespoons or ½ pint or 8 fluid ounces

2 cups = 1 pint or 16 fluid ounces

1 quart = 2 pints or 4 cups or 32 fluid ounces

1 gallon = 4 quarts or 8 pints or 16 cups or 128 fluid ounces

Resources

All the nonperishable foods used in this cookbook, such as stevia, xylitol, brown rice syrup, and cardia salt are sold in health food stores, or may be ordered from:

Whitaker Wellness Institute
4321 Birch Street
Newport Beach, CA 92660
800-810-6655
www.whitakerwellness.com

Mother's Market
225 East 17th Street
Costa Mesa, CA 92627
800-595-MOMS
949-631-4741
www.mothersmarket.com

About the
Whitaker Wellness Institute

Founded in 1979 by Julian Whitaker, M.D., the Whitaker Wellness Institute is one of the oldest and most respected alternative medicine clinics in the United States. More than thirty thousand patients from all over the world have come to the clinic seeking treatment for diabetes and other diseases with safe, proven therapies that are ignored by conventional physicians.

Most patients who come to the clinic participate in the one-, two-, or three-week Back to Health Program. This program involves an extensive medical evaluation, complete laboratory blood workup, and appropriate diagnostic testing. Patients are then prescribed a personalized program of nutritional supplements, an individualized exercise program, and a therapeutic diet.

During their stay at the clinic, patients attend informative, hands-on workshops, including nutrition lectures and cooking demonstrations. They participate in guided exercise sessions and eat delicious, healthful meals prepared by our gourmet chef. They also enjoy the support and guidance of our caring, professional staff as well as the encouragement and camaraderie of their fellow patients.

Patients may also be treated with leading-edge therapies to address diabetic complications. These include EECP (Enhanced External Counter-Pulsation) to enhance circulation, relieve angina, and improve diabetic neuropathy; hyperbaric oxygen therapy, which floods the cells with oxygen and is especially beneficial for nonhealing diabetic ulcers, neuropathy, and retinopathy; and intravenous therapies such as EDTA chelation to facilitate the healing of diabetic ulcers, or nutrients that reverse the progression of diabetic retinopathy.

For more information contact the Whitaker Wellness Institute:

Whitaker Wellness Institute
4321 Birch Street
Newport Beach, CA 92660
800-488-1500
whitakerwellness.com

About *Health & Healing*

Since 1991, Dr. Whitaker's monthly newsletter *Health & Healing* has reached millions of readers, providing them with safe, natural solutions to a multitude of health problems. Dr. Whitaker has been a driving force in alternative medicine for the past twenty-five years. In addition to informing his readers about effective new therapies, he also tirelessly crusades for medical freedom. *Health & Healing* was recently rated one of the top ten health newsletters in the country by *Time* magazine.

For information on *Health & Healing,* contact:

Phillips Health
800-539-8219
www.drwhitaker.com

Index